NURSING HISTORY REVIEW

OFFICIAL JOURNAL OF
THE AMERICAN ASSOCIATION FOR THE HISTORY OF NURSING

ISSN 1062-8061   2000 • Volume 8

CONTENTS

Springer Publishing Company • New York

EDITOR'S NOTE

We wish to correct two errors found in Volume 7. In the opening paragraph of the article, "Vivian Bullwinkle: Survivor of the 1942 Massacre of Australian Nurses," Matron Paschke was incorrectly identified as a survivor of the war. In fact, she drowned in February 1942 during the sinking of the S.S. Vyner Brooke. In the same article, another nurse's name was misspelled. It should read Wilma Oram. The authors regret these errors.

Cover photo: Graduate nurse preparing a clysis, Philadelphia General Hospital, Circa 1900 (by Permission of the Center for The Study of The History of Nursing, School of Nursing, University of Pennsylvania).

Nursing History Review is published annually for the American Association for the History of Nursing, Inc., by Springer Publishing Company, Inc., New York.

Business office: All business correspondence, including subscriptions, renewals, advertising, and address changes, should be sent to Springer Publishing Company, 536 Broadway, New York, NY 10012–3955.

Editorial offices: Submit six copies of the manuscript for publication. Submissions and editorial correspondence should be directed to Joan E. Lynaugh, Editor, *Nursing History Review,* University of Pennsylvania, 420 Guardian Drive, Room 307, Philadelphia, PA 19104-6096. See *Guidelines for Contributors* on the inside back cover for further details.

Members of the American Association for the History of Nursing, Inc. (AAHN) receive *Nursing History Review* on payment of annual membership dues. Applications and other correspondence relating to AAHN membership should be directed to Janet L. Fickeissen, Executive Secretary, American Association for the History of Nursing, Inc., P.O. Box 175, Lonoka Harbor, NJ 08734-0175

Subscription rates: Volume 8, 2000. For institutions: $68/1 year, $120/2 years. For individuals: $36/1 year, $66/2 years. Outside the United States—for institutions: $80/1 year, $140/2 years; for individuals: $43/1 year, $77/2 years. Air ship available: $12/year. Payment must be made in U.S. dollars through a U.S. bank. Make checks payable to Springer Publishing Company.

Indexes/abstracts of articles for this journal appear in *CINAHL® print & database, Current Contents/Social & Behavioral Sciences, Social Sciences Citation Index, Research Alert, RNdex, Index Medicus/MEDLINE, Historical Abstracts, America: History of Life.*

Postmaster: Send address changes to Springer Publishing Company, Inc., 536 Broadway, New York, NY 10012–3955.

ISSN 1062-8061

ISBN 0-8261-1317-6

American Association for the History of Nursing, Inc.

EDITORIAL

Some time ago, a colleague asked me to write a short statement discussing the place of historical research in the contemporary nursing research scene. I happily filled her request, citing the intellectual and professional enrichment history offers to nursing. I commented on the complementary explanatory power of history in a field dominated by research grounded in the scientific method. When I was finished, I filed the paper in my computer under the title "history is good." A slightly whimsical title, I admit. It reflects the frequency with which I am asked to defend history as an appropriate subject for research in nursing. Thinking it over, however, I think we should also ask ourselves "is our history really good?" By this I mean is the history we write good enough to read for fun? Most of us who were educated as health professionals learned to describe our findings using an economy of words yielding an almost terse style. We wrote in the passive voice, never in the first person, and maybe we were even encouraged to use professional and technical jargon. Speaking from experience, I believe converting one's style from writing this way to writing narrative is very difficult. It is also absolutely essential to making history "really good." Now, I don't mean to imply that nurses who do history are the only historians with this difficulty. In fact, academics are rather often accused of deliberately making the obvious obscure. Sometimes it seems we are striving for dullness. But the history of nursing is full of unique and fascinating events and people; our subject is not dull. I think the task of writing is to make the narrative live for the reader in the same way it thrills us as we discover it. Good history tells the whole story, usually in chronological fashion with a beginning, middle, and end. It is a big challenge to set the time, get the facts right and in their proper context, and to do it in such a way that the reader clings to the story. History is a story after all, and we want our stories to be remembered. We want them to affect how others understand the past and the present. Historian David Kennedy urges us to approach our history as we would write a novel.[1] Our historical figures are characters, he argues; they deserve description and life on our pages. Their conflicts need explication and interpretation. Change occurs and issues do or do not get resolved. The real history of nursing written in real-life terms will keep the reader in thrall. I make no claim that this is easy or that I can do it myself most of the time. I do know that the best history I read is written to attract and hold the reader and one of the joys of being your editor is my frequent opportunity to open mail containing "really good" history.

Note

[1]David Kennedy, "The Art of the Tale: Story-Telling and History Teaching," *Reviews in American History* (Baltimore: The Johns Hopkins University Press, 1998) 462-473.

JOAN E. LYNAUGH

Center for the Study of the History of Nursing
University of Pennsylvania

ARTICLES

The Physician's Eyes
American Nursing and the Diagnostic Revolution in Medicine

MARGARETE SANDELOWSKI

Department of Women's and Children's Health
University of North Carolina at Chapel Hill

(The) Nurse Should Be the Doctor's Eyes in His Absence[1]

The emergence of trained nursing in the United States in the 1870s and its capture[2] in hospitals by the 1930s did not merely coincide with the diagnostic revolution that fundamentally transformed American medicine in this period; they were tightly linked. During this time, hospitals were increasingly sold to potential patients as sites for the sympathetic and scientific care embodied in the new trained nurse and the new diagnostic technology housed there. Although barely (if at all) mentioned in histories of medical technology and hospitals, nurses were more than footnotes in the story of how technologically mediated diagnosis became a distinguishing feature of medical practice and hospital care. Nurses played a crucial role in this transformation, sharing with physicians the use of such new devices as the thermometer and often performing much of the physical, mental, and "sentimental"[3] labor engendered by x-ray and laboratory tests. Nurses made hospitals more hospitable, not only to patients but also to the new devices and device-mediated techniques that became the sine qua non of medical practice. In this article I focus on nursing and the new diagnostic technology in the formative years—from 1873 to the early 1930s—of both modern American nursing and technologically mediated medical diagnosis. I use the term technology to refer not only to devices but also to the social interactions, divisions of labor, and human purposes around these devices.

The Diagnostic Revolution in Medicine

Historians of medicine and medical technology have emphasized the enormous impact on medicine of the introduction of such sense-extending devices

Nursing History Review 8 (2000): 3-38. A publication of the American Association for the History of Nursing. Copyright © 2000 Springer Publishing Company.

as the stethoscope, ophthalmoscope, laryngoscope, and fluoroscope and of such device-mediated techniques to measure, monitor, analyze, and record body functions as clinical thermometry, electrocardiography, and chemical assays of urine, blood, and other body fluids. They also have described the initial reluctance many physicians expressed toward using them.[4] The new diagnostic technology enhanced physicians' abilities to investigate and diagnose disease and their prestige as the preeminent practitioners of science. Indeed, physicians derived much of their cultural authority from their association with a technology that was seen to embody science.[5]

However, physicians feared not only "losing touch"[6] with patients (in the dual senses of losing contact with them and losing the skill of "digital observation"[7]) but also losing their authority and exclusive claim to the knowledge and skill that using this technology required and the knowledge about disease it offered. Physicians were concerned that reliance on technology would undermine their efforts to practice and to present medicine as an intellectual and independent, as opposed to manual and collaborative, pursuit. In the early 19th century, physicians associated technology with the manual labor, instrumentation, and barbarities of surgeons from whom they were eager to disassociate themselves. By the end of that century, however, physicians were recognizing that the new diagnostic devices, like surgical instruments, allowed physicians not only to improve medical practice and advance medical science but also to be seen as actively and concretely doing something to earn the social standing, authority, and remuneration they sought.

Eager to "purge subjectivity"[8] from, and to incorporate science into, the practice of medicine, physicians increasingly relied on what they perceived as objective instrument- or machine-generated information. They became less comfortable with patient descriptions and their own unaided senses as the sole or even primary basis for diagnosis. However, in the process of augmenting their diagnostic power and cultural authority the new technology had the effect of separating physicians from their patients. Physicians were socially separated from patients by acquiring increasingly specialized and arcane knowledge not readily accessible to anyone but themselves. What the doctor heard and saw through the magic and science of the stethoscope and microscope could not easily be heard, seen, or understood by others. Physicians' new knowledge, which set them apart from and elevated them above patients and other professional competitors seeking access to the patient's bedside, constituted an advantageous separation.

Yet, generalist physicians were also physically separated from patients as medical diagnosis was increasingly accomplished at a distance from the patient and through the efforts of specialists, including other physicians, nurses, and technicians. For example, although the stethoscope brought physicians closer to patients' bodies than they had been, it also maintained a space between the patient's body and the physician's ear. Rene Laennec, the inventor of "mediate auscultation"[9] via the stethoscope in the early 19th century, was reportedly motivated by the desire not only to hear the sounds of body organs but also to avoid the close physical contact with patients that placing an ear to the body entailed but which social mores made suspect. The microscope, in turn, permitted diagnosis to occur without any patient present at all. And, laboratory and x-ray diagnosis increasingly required what the general physician in practice typically or often did not have, namely, the time and expertise of specialists to conduct these tests and to interpret their results.

Historians have described and even glorified physicians' relations to the new diagnostic technology, but its relations to nursing remain virtually unexplored. Did the technology play as central a role in redefining nursing as it did in redefining medicine? That is, was the diagnostic revolution as revolutionary for nursing? While diagnosis, in some form, had always been central to medical practice and the physician-patient relationship, was it as critical to nursing practice and the nurse–patient relationship even in the new era of diagnosis? What did nurses gain and lose with the advent of new diagnostic techniques? What were nursing's concerns around these techniques? What did nurses contribute to the diagnostic revolution in medicine and what, in turn, were the immediate and long-term effects of this revolution on nursing?

I begin to address these questions here. I focus on what nurses and physicians perceived as one of the most essential functions of the nurse, namely, to serve as the physician's eyes. Physicians appropriated nurses' eyes as proxies for their own even as they were appropriating nurses' hands to carry out patient care. Nurses were trained and expected to collect, record, and interpret information vital to the diagnosis—and, therefore, to the treatment and prognosis of disease under the putatively watchful eyes of physicians, without making any claims to participating in diagnosis. The trained nurse's eyes were, if not the first, then the most critical instruments in physicians' new diagnostic armamentarium.

Trained Nursing and the Trained Senses

In the formative years of American-trained nursing, nursing observation was largely an embodied relation with patients in which nurses relied on their trained senses of sight, touch, and smell. Indeed, the "trained nurse" (typically conceived and, therefore, referred to here as female) was distinguished from other female caregivers, in part, by the "trained senses" she directed toward the "close observation" that promised to elevate nursing above "mechanical, routine, nonintelligent practice and place it upon a scientific, professional basis."[10] In contrast to the behaviorist cast the idea had in the 1920s and 1930s, the psychodynamic and interpersonal casts it acquired after World War II (WWII), and the phenomenological and narrative casts it has today, knowing the patient[11] used to mean knowing the patient largely in the flesh. Nursing was primarily an intimate corporeal relation involving the physical bodies of patients and the physical senses and ministrations of nurses. Listening to patients, in the sense of eliciting and interpreting their stories to know them by heart—as well as by sight, smell, and touch—had yet to become a prevailing and integral part of the rhetoric or fabric of the nurse–patient relationship.[12] Indeed, Florence Nightingale viewed too much talking on the part of both patients and nurses as physically taxing and, therefore, as indicative of poor nursing practice.

FLORENCE NIGHTINGALE AND THE OBSERVATION OF THE SICK

Nightingale had established observation as the habit and faculty that enhanced the utility of and legitimized the need for trained nurses. Nightingale believed that a woman who could not cultivate this habit ought to abandon the pursuit of nursing, even though she might be kind. In 1860 in the classic primer *Notes on Nursing,* she instructed:

> The most important practical lesson that can be given to nurses is to teach them what to observe—how to observe—what symptoms indicate improvement—what the reverse—which are of importance—which are of none—which are the evidence of neglect—and of what kind of neglect.[13]

For Nightingale, acquiring the habit and faculty of observation was no simple feat. Speaking " the whole truth and nothing but the truth "—whether in court or at the bedside—required "many faculties combined of observation and memory."[14] There was no more "final proof"[15] in the fact that a person had told the same story many times than there was in the fact that one story had been corroborated by many people. Nightingale had no patience with nurses who, albeit unknowingly, imparted false information about patients to physicians. False information often resulted from asking the wrong (that is, "leading" instead of "pointed")[16] questions.

Nightingale carved out an essential role for nursing in the diagnosis and treatment of conditions leading to poor health and sickness, even as physicians were increasingly claiming diagnosis and treatment exclusively for themselves. Moreover, in an era when most physicians were just beginning to understand the specific etiologies of disease and the importance of clearly differentiating one disease or disorder from another, and to adopt the view that specific treatments should be matched to specific diagnoses,[17] Nightingale's ideal nurse was an expert in a kind of differential diagnosis not heretofore practiced by either nurses or physicians. This nurse was able to discriminate among symptoms deriving from disease itself, from the therapies chosen to treat these diseases, from deficiencies in the patient's life circumstances that might have initially contributed to the disease, and most important, from failures of the nurse "to put the patient in the best condition for nature to act upon him."[18] The trained nurse could differentiate, for example, among defects in cooking, choice of diet, choice of hours for taking food, and in the appetite as causes of "want of nutrition"[19] in the patient. The trained nurse also understood that each of these defects, in turn, required different remedies. The remedy for the first defect was to cook better, for the second was to make other choices in diet, for the third was to offer patients food when they wanted it, and for the fourth was to show patients what they liked.[20]

Nightingale admired nurses who had developed a precision of eye virtually equal to the measuring glass, although she maintained that nurses' eyes could not fully substitute for the accuracy of this device. An observant nurse could tell at a glance how many ounces of food her patient had consumed, even if the amount was very small. Nurses also had to learn the "physiognomy,"[21] or look, of various diseases and how they appeared in combination with the looks of individual patients. Nightingale promoted nursing observation as the artful and idiographic corrective to the scientific "averages" that threatened to seduce nurses away from "minute observation"[22] and physicians away from the particularities and peculiarities of individual cases.

In summary, Nightingale's nurse cultivated the habit and faculty of observation to achieve the good nursing care upon which good medical care depended. In the days before the development of specific pharmacologic agents or public health measures targeted directly at the causes of disease and before the refinement of aseptic surgical techniques, medical care often entailed little else but nursing care. The trained nurse had knowledge only nurses could possess by virtue of their constant presence at the bedside, and it was this very privileged knowledge that physicians needed for accurate assessment and management of patient conditions. Nightingale's observant nurse not only enhanced the comfort and promoted the health of her patients, but she often also saved their lives and saved the day for physicians who might otherwise be misled by the limited information available to them from their abbreviated contacts with patients.

AMERICAN TRAINED NURSING AND THE POWERS OF OBSERVATION

Nightingale's instructions concerning observation and its importance in nursing and medical practice were incorporated and developed in the earliest lectures to and instructional texts for American students of nursing.[23] American instructors also pointed to observation as a critical feature distinguishing trained nursing from uneducated womanly ministrations to the sick. They emphasized the value of trained nursing and the shortcomings of medicine by repeatedly reminding students that it was nurses who provided accurate descriptions of patient conditions "to those who have had no opportunity for persistent observation."[24] The physician was completely dependent on the nurse for what only she could know and for what he had to know. As Clara S. Weeks, the author of one of the most influential early textbooks of nursing, concluded:

> The nurse, who is with her patient constantly, has, if she knows how to make use of it, a much better opportunity of becoming acquainted with his real condition than the physician, who only spends half an hour with him occasionally.[25]

Indeed, according to Weeks, the "very excitement"[26] of (or agitation caused by) the physician's visit often so altered patients' conditions that they might look better or worse to the visiting physician than they really were. In addition, patients often told nurses things they did not tell their doctors. Nursing observation was especially crucial in the cases of infants, delirious patients, and others who could not or ought not—in order to conserve their energy—speak for themselves. The trained nurse was the physician's eyes, but she did not so much extend a largely sighted physician as a virtually blind one. Indeed, he saw very little without her.

Authors, such as Weeks, who sought to establish nursing as a valued profession for women, recurringly reminded students of nursing of the responsibility and power that lay in the nurse's eyes and in the constancy of her vigilance at the bedside. The physician depended on the nurse's "powers of observation"[27] and in that dependence lay her professional power. Accordingly, nurses were taught to take careful notice of their patients and the conditions surrounding them. Didactic texts emphasized the physical condition of the patient, physical manifestations indicating aberrant mental states, and the physical environment of the sick room. Nightingale's admonition to nurses to learn the laws of health and to observe the total life circumstances of their patients could be more closely adhered to in home and public health nursing, where nurses had the opportunity to see the larger family and other social circumstances of their patients that contributed to ill health. In the hospital, however, nurses were confined largely to observations of the physical and proximate causes of disease and discomfort, that is, to what could be immediately seen, felt, smelled, or heard from outside the body and to such factors in the physical environment as ventilation, lighting, and noise.

Nurses' "relation to symptomatology"[28] was a major topic of instruction from the earliest days of trained nursing. Nurses were taught to differentiate between subjective and objective symptoms, between symptoms and signs, between real and feigned symptoms, between leading and misleading symptoms, and between symptoms and signs significant for nursing care and those significant for medical care. They were to note and record the degree, character, duration, frequency, time of occurrence, apparent cause, modification, and significance of an array of symptoms and signs, such as pain, palpitation, dyspnea, cough, expectoration, and vomiting. Nurses were to appraise the condition of every visible portion of the body, using parameters appropriate for that part. For example, they were to observe the color, volume, degree of moisture, coating, markings, motion, and manner of protrusion of the tongue. They were to note the rate, volume, strength, rhythm, and tension of the pulse.[29] Before technological intrusions into the living body were routine in clinical practice, learning the subtleties of symptomatology and of patient expression, posture, mood, and temperament was especially critical. What could be discerned from the outside comprised virtually all the information available to the general nursing or medical practitioner.

Practicing close observation entailed not only cultivating the sensory faculties but also understanding and managing its effect on patients. Being under the constant scrutiny of professional strangers, whether in the home or hospital, was new to patients unused to either trained nursing in the home or to hospital care. While being looked after was likely comforting to most patients, being looked at could be disturbing and even result in error. Nurses were admonished not to let patients know they were being observed because this could generate misleading symptoms.[30] Nurses learned to observe patients while they were ministering to their needs; that is, they learned to take opportunities, such as the bath, to note conditions of the body. They also learned to observe one patient while caring for another. Nurse trainee Mary Clymer noted the difficulty she had "trying to have my eyes in 13 while my hands make a bed in 11."[31]

In short, the close observation expected of the trained nurse required knowledge of symptoms and signs and their various relations to disease, treatment, and environmental conditions, the cultivation of all the nurse's senses with an emphasis on the practiced and disciplined eye, savvy in patient relations, and the ability to communicate and increasingly record observations in a manner likely to be of most use to both patient and physician. If the key to good nursing was observation, the key to accurate medical diagnosis and patient recovery was the close observation of the trained nurse. The trained nurse was to be all-seeing: to take all of the "visual opportunities"[32] available to her and to maintain "visual control"[33] of her patients and the sick room. Except for the candle, gas, stopwatch (to count the pulse), and, later, electric light, nursing observation in the late 19th century was largely an in-the-flesh practice unmediated by technological devices.[34]

The Instrumental Eye

While nurses were learning the importance of observing the sick, medical practice in the latter decades of the 19th, and early decades of the 20th, century increasingly involved new technological means of observing living patients, of looking into and through them in addition to looking at and over them. From the middle of the 19th century, physical diagnosis with and without sense-extending devices such as the stethoscope increasingly prevailed. After 1900 the primacy and value of physical diagnosis were increasingly challenged by the x-ray and the analytic, graphic, and quantitative techniques of laboratory diagnosis, electrocardiography, and sphygmomanometry.[35] In order to harness the benefits of this new technology, physicians had to share its use with nurses (and, eventually, also with a host of new technicians whose jobs were created in response to it). These new "instruments of precision"[36] and symbols of medical science not only complicated the nurse's work but also blurred the boundary line between nursing and medical practice.

CLINICAL THERMOMETRY
Clinical thermometry became part of American medical practice in the latter part of the 19th century. Although the mercury thermometer had been

invented early in the 18th century, its initial design made it impractical as a clinical tool. Thermometers were originally rather large devices, about a foot long and bent at a right angle, which had to be carried in a holster under the arm, much as "one might carry a gun."[37] Moreover, because thermometers did not maintain temperature readings at their maximum level once they were removed from the body, physicians had to read them while they were still placed against the body. The invention of portable and self-registering devices that maintained the temperature at its maximum reading after removal from the body, the 1871 translation of Carl Wunderlich's scientific treatise on medical thermometry,[38] and the 1873 translation of Edouard Seguin's manual on medical and family thermometry,[39] contributed to the virtually complete replacement in American clinical practice, by the end of the 19th century, of the hand with the thermometer to discern patient temperature. The glass or metal thermometer replaced the "hand-thermometer,"[40] or the hand, as the thermometer.

In contrast to other diagnostic devices, such as the stethoscope, laryngoscope, and microscope, which nurses assisted physicians in using and/ or only occasionally used themselves, the direct use of the thermometer was soon delegated to nurses. Indeed, nurses became the most likely and frequent users of this device, charged with taking temperatures in the physician's absence and with maintaining the thermometers themselves. The thermometer was rather quickly incorporated into routine nursing practice and, almost as quickly, came to be associated with, and even to represent, nursing. The earliest American textbooks of nursing and lecture notes indicate that nurses were expected to use the thermometer in their daily practice, that is, at the very least, to take and record the temperature.[41] Advertisements for preprinted blank temperature. charts appear in the back of texts written for nurses, indicating that nurses were responsible for maintaining legible records of patients' temperatures.[42] The thermometer was a prominent feature of what nurses, physicians, and advertisers considered to be part of the nurse's "uniform," "armamentarium," "chatelaine," and "nurse's case."[43] Companies manufacturing thermometers marketed them directly to nurses and as suitable gifts for nurses (see Figure 1).[44] Early popular verbal and pictorial depictions of nursing, as well as advertisements for nursing itself, often presented the nurse with a "thermometer in her hand"[45] The thermometer was soon even incorporated into the image nurses had of themselves and their functions. In her widely read 1893 textbook on nursing, Isabel Hampton encouraged the nurse to think of herself as the "ward thermometer and barometer (alert for) any change in the ward atmosphere."[46] Nurses not only used thermometers; they were thermometers.

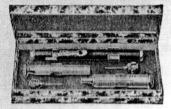
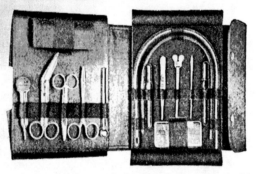
Figure 1. Becton, Dickinson ad marketing thermometers as suitable gifts for nurses.

Thermometry was depicted also as a womanly "handicraft,"[47] and the thermometer itself was depicted as a means "second to none"[48] in the practice of the womanly arts of mothering and nursing. Seguin, who popularized "family thermometry," viewed the handling and intelligent reading of the thermometer and the accurate recording of the temperature as necessary to learning the "ABC of motherhood."[49] The thermometer was necessary also to "that part of nursing which mainly consists in spying the subtle and bold invasion of disease, and of measuring . . . its deadly strides into the vitals of the innocent."[50] Women were the sentries who would be first to detect and "measure the strength of the enemy on the stem of [their] thermometers."[51]

The earliest instructions that nurses received about the thermometer show varying detail and increasing complexity, with information ranging from the procedural—that is, how to take, read, and record the temperature in adults and children—to the scientific—that is, the theoretical basis for clinical thermometry and the meaning of various temperatures and temperature profiles in the progression of disease. In Bellevue Hospital's 1878 *Manual of Nursing*, only one paragraph on the thermometer appears at the end of the book as an addendum, and it contains information on how to take an oral temperature, a reference to axillary and rectal temperatures, and what the normal axillary temperature is.[52] The Connecticut Training School's *Handbook of Nursing*, published in 1879, contains somewhat more information and a reference to Seguin's work.[53]

Fourteen years later, in 1893, in the first edition of *Nursing*,[54] Hampton devoted a chapter to temperature, linking variations in temperature to variations in pulse and respiration, and differentiating normal from abnormal temperatures, and addressing diurnal variations in temperature and factors (such as the placement of thermometers and the temperature and nature of foods) that could raise or lower temperature. Hampton classified temperatures, ranging from the "temperature of collapse" at 95°–97°F to "hyperpyrexia"[55] at over 105°F, and she differentiated among continuous, intermittent, and remittent fevers. She included "specimen charts"[56] showing temperature, pulse, and respiration in typhoid fever, pneumonia, and malaria. Hampton taught nurses how to convert Fahrenheit to Centigrade and Centigrade to Fahrenheit temperatures, how to test a thermometer for accuracy, how to take mouth, axillary, and rectal temperatures, and how to clean and store thermometers. Reprising concerns raised by physicians about the dangers of substituting instruments for the trained senses of the clinician, Hampton advised nurses not to rely solely on the thermometer. Even though ascertaining temperature by touch alone could be highly misleading (as skin temperature was not a reliable indicator of body temperature), touching the patient was still an essential component of nursing observation that allowed the detection of conditions that might go unnoticed without it.

Didactic instructions for nurses concerning thermometry became more detailed over the years, providing more information on the scientific basis for clinical thermometry and its relation to the diagnosis and course of disease and detection of patient responses to treatment. Since many so-called medical treatments entailed nothing but nursing care (as in "fever" nursing[57]), the thermometer was as much an instrument of nursing—assisting the nurse to evaluate the effectiveness of her ministrations—as it was an instrument of medicine. As Bertha Harmer noted in the first edition in 1922 of probably the most widely read series of textbooks of nursing,[58] it was not enough for the nurse merely to be able to take the temperature. She had to know what caused various temperatures to occur and the nursing measures that would lower and raise temperature to normal levels. The nurse did not merely take the temperature; she used the thermometer to diagnose, monitor, and rediagnose patient conditions.

As thermometry became routine in clinical practice and virtually the sole province—in the hospital—of the nurse, instructional texts for nursing included increasingly more information on "making temperature taking safe."[59] The "safety work"[60] of clinical thermometry included the maintenance and disinfection of thermometers, ensuring the accuracy of thermometer readings, and preventing harm to patients. Both instructional texts teaching nurses about thermometers and advertising texts promoting the sales of competing brands of thermometers indicate that breakage was a constant concern.[61] Nurses considered themselves fortunate if they were not required to pay for the thermometers they broke.[62] Since the same thermometer typically had to be shared among patients, nurses were also increasingly concerned with the best methods to clean thermometers. Clinical thermometry was one of the earliest focal points of scientific investigation by nurses as they evaluated the effectiveness of various procedures for disinfection of thermometers. Most notable in this area of research was the 1929. Martha E. Erdmann and Margaret Welsh report of the studies in thermometer technique they had conducted between 1927 and 1928.[63]

The safety work of clinical thermometry also included preventing situations likely to cause injury to patients from broken thermometers or from false temperature readings. Nurses were cautioned about hysterical or malingering patients who deliberately sought to elevate temperature readings by placing the thermometer against something hot while the nurse was not looking. There were also other uncooperative patients who did not or could not keep the thermometer in place for the length of time required to register its maximum reading. Nurses were warned never to leave patients unattended with thermometers in place unless they were certain that it was safe to leave a patient unsupervised or that the patient was physically able, or could be trusted, to be left alone.[64] Although clinical thermometry did not create the view that patients were themselves often unreliable partners in restoring them back to health, it reinforced and extended the view of thermometry as a practice that depended on the cooperation of the patient.

Clinical thermometry served also to influence the aesthetics of nursing (and of hospital nursing, in particular), affecting the order and structure of work on the ward and the appearance of nursing care. As physicians became more interested in the scientific investigation of disease and in establishing patterns of temperature in various diseases, they ordered temperatures to be taken more frequently. Whereas temperatures might have initially been taken once or twice a day, increasingly, temperatures had to be taken four or more times in a 24-hour period. Under ideal conditions, thermometers required 3–5 minutes to register temperature in the mouth but up to 15 minutes to register temperature in the axilla, often a preferred mode of taking the temperature. Moreover, the normal diurnal variations in temperature made it necessary to take temperatures at times when body temperature tended to be at its lowest and highest levels. Physicians also expected all temperatures to be taken and recorded before their scheduled morning and/or evening rounds. Accordingly, the practice soon arose of assigning one nurse—the "temperature nurse"[65]—to take and record all the temperatures on a ward. This early manifestation of functional nursing—that is, giving one task to one nurse for her to complete on all patients—stood in sharp contrast to the home or private duty model of nursing where one nurse provided all the care that one patient required. The "temperature nurse" was a new factor that detracted from the exclusivity of the traditional nurse–patient relationship.

Thermometers also figured prominently in the development of specialized equipment trays that became a characteristic feature of nursing care. These trays were a means for the nurse to be efficient and organized in gathering and arranging the materials needed to conduct procedures at the bedside and to give a finished appearance to her work. In instructional and advice literature concerning the thermometer and other trays, nurses were told to consider not only functionality and safety in their work but also symmetry and neatness in presenting equipment to patients and physicians. Indeed, symmetry and neatness were critical features of the rotating system nurses used to distinguish between clean and dirty thermometers and, thereby, to prevent inadvertently using a dirty thermometer.[66]

In summary, from the beginning of American trained nursing the thermometer became both fact and symbol of nursing practice. The thermometer was an instrument that helped the nurse to diagnose and monitor patient conditions and to detect defects in nursing and medical care. As an instrument increasingly linked in professional, popular, and advertising literature with nurses, the thermometer represented both the precision of science and the ministrations of the trained nursing. Moreover, the thermometer forged a link between nursing and technology, whereby nurses came to understand themselves not only as users of scientific instruments but also as functioning like them.

(STETHO)SCOPIC EXAMINATIONS

In the case of the thermometer the practice of taking and recording the temperature eventually fell to the woman or nurse in the home and to the nurse in the hospital. In contrast, scopic examinations, or physical examinations conducted with such eye- and ear-extending instruments as ophthalmoscopes, laryngoscopes, and stethoscopes, remained largely in the physician's domain through the 1930s. If nurses participated in scopic examinations at all, it was primarily to hold patients in position for the examination, to ensure their cooperation, and to see to it that the proper equipment was at the physician's hand.[67]

Nurses' use of the stethoscope in this period was confined largely to listening to the fetal heart, although the practice of regular fetal auscultation, conducted with increasing frequency as labor progressed to delivery, had yet to become standard obstetric practice.[68] Nurses sometimes also used stethoscopes to take blood pressure, but taking the blood pressure did not become part of routine nursing practice until the 1930s. Nurses were instructed about blood pressure, but didactic literature and procedure manuals directed toward them indicate that taking the blood pressure was not something they were expected to do at all or on a regular basis.[69] Although there were physicians in the first decade of the 20th century who still viewed blood pressure measurement as a dangerous substitute for digital observation (or palpation) of the pulse,[70] blood pressure was typically conceived as a component of the physical examination of patients that only physicians conducted.

Moreover, in contrast to clinical thermometry, the labor involved in scopic examinations was not so easily divided and delegated. One user could not simply take and record scopically derived information for another user to interpret as these instruments did not permanently register any number or graphic analogue to the temperature. Unlike the temperature scale, which anyone with reasonable visual acuity could see on a thermometer, the use of scopic devices depended on having the specialized scientific knowledge and perceptual skill to see or hear device-mediated objects and sounds, an interpretive skill apart from the skill of interpreting what these objects and sounds meant for the diagnosis of disease.

Because these instruments entailed interpretive skills that were taught exclusively to physicians, they remained outside of the sphere of the nurse. In addition, the belief seemed to prevail that scopic examinations were not appropriate for nurses to learn, as they were at the heart of the diagnostic encounter between physician and patient. One physician reported in 1888 being rebuked for teaching a nurse stethoscopic examination of the chest to detect heart complications in a case of rheumatism. Nurses, he was warned, would get into trouble for having "too much knowledge for a nurse."[71] The stethoscope, especially, seemed to symbolize medicine and the art and new science of physical diagnosis, much as the thermometer became a symbol of nursing.[72]

X-RAY AND LABORATORY DIAGNOSIS

In the first 3 decades of the 20th century, patients were increasingly subjected to x-ray and laboratory examinations to diagnose and monitor their ailments or to detect disease that had not as yet produced any discernible ailments. In this period, patients entered hospitals not only to receive medical treatment and nursing care for illness or injury but also to find out whether and why they were sick. Moreover, x-ray and laboratory tests were increasingly used to assign and confirm diagnoses already made and as ritual screening components of hospitalization. By the 1930s, being admitted to a hospital entailed having an x-ray taken, having blood drawn, and providing a urine sample.[73] X-ray and laboratory technology embodied the new scientific hospital, and x-ray and laboratory units and equipment were prominently featured in annual reports and other materials promoting hospitals.[74]

As a consequence of their increasing reliance on x-ray and laboratory testing, physicians in general practice became increasingly dependent on specialist physicians, nurses, and others to use this technology. Roentgenographic and laboratory tests exemplified, perhaps more than any other technological innovations, the extent to which diagnosis became an interdependent and collaborative process involving physicians, nurses, technicians, and patients, rather than a discrete moment in exclusively physician time. Unlike clinical thermometry and scopic examinations, these tests entailed many activities that could be demarcated from each other and then delegated. Exactly what components of this new diagnostic work nurses performed depended on such factors as the extent of x-ray and laboratory testing conducted in the hospitals in which they worked and the availability of house physicians, specialist physicians, and technicians to do the work. For example, smaller hospitals typically offered less extensive in-house testing, but they also had fewer or no house physicians or other ancillary personnel to do this work. Shortages of personnel were especially acute after World War I (WWI).

Accordingly, nurses' work in x-ray and laboratory diagnosis variously included the before, during, and after care of equipment and of patients at the bedside or in the units in which the tests were conducted, the transportation of patients to these units, the collection, labeling, storing, and delivery of specimens, the creation and maintenance of written records of these examinations, and/or the conduct of the examinations themselves. Urinometers to measure the specific gravity of urine, litmus paper to determine its pH, and other devices to measure albumin and sugar were part of the nurse's outfit and responsibilities from the earliest days of trained nursing.[75] Nurses also performed a promotional function for hospitals by taking visitors (during annual events such as Hospital Day) on tours through laboratory and x-ray units and showing off the new scientific equipment housed there.[76]

In addition to carrying out the various tasks associated with x-ray and laboratory testing on the unit, nurses were employed in x-ray and laboratory departments themselves as roentgen assistants, administering barium for fluoroscopic examinations of the gastrointestinal tract (see Figure 2) and maintaining records. Nurses were also employed as x-ray technicians and microscopists in hospitals and physicians' offices, obtaining and developing x-ray pictures and conducting chemical assays of blood, urine, sputum, and other specimens. As students, nurses were rotated through x-ray and laboratory departments and had available to them elective training in x-ray or laboratory work in their last year of school and in postgraduate courses.[77]

There were both nurses and physicians who promoted x-ray and laboratory work as nursing specialties. Nurses advocating nurse specialization saw this work as an opportunity to gain knowledge and skills that would make them more marketable to physicians and hospitals. In an era when most nursing positions in hospitals were still filled by student nurses and when graduate nurses were increasingly competing with each other for decreasing positions in the home and in public health, the "needy"[78] x-ray and laboratory fields offered employment to the equally needy graduate nurse. The routinization of x-ray

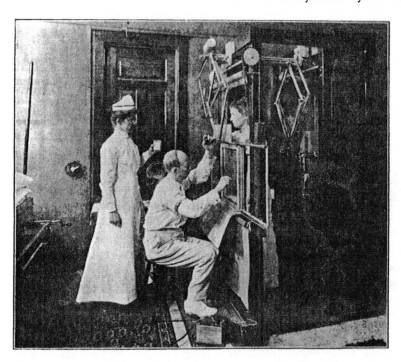

Figure 2. A nurse employed in an x-ray department.

and laboratory diagnosis also legitimized the need for more science education in nursing curricula to make nurses more able assistants. The work that this new kind of diagnosis generated made knowledge of anatomy, physiology, physics, chemistry, and bacteriology even more essential. Moreover, by virtue of the association of x-ray and laboratory technology with the much revered science, nurses who were knowledgeable in these fields could further differentiate themselves not only from untrained nurses but also from the trained nurses who knew nothing of these fields. Both nurse and physician advocates of nursing specialization in these fields promoted roentgen and laboratory work as especially fitting for nurses showing a "scientific turn of mind."[79]

For nurse and physician proponents of nurse specialization in x-ray and laboratory work these fields offered an interesting departure from and often better working conditions than bedside nursing.[80] They argued that the hours of work were generally more regular and convenient, that the pay was sometimes better, and that the nurse won a reprieve from the daily complexities and physical exertions of caring for sick people that tended to shorten her working life. Yet, although a departure from traditional bedside nursing, the work permitted the nurse to draw from her nursing background to alleviate the discomfort and fear that patients, especially children, experienced as they encountered these strange new tests.

Indeed, as nurse advocates proposed, this work demanded not only the technical skills associated with applying the technology but also the skills of the trained nurse in managing patients' emotions and in protecting the privacy these tests often threatened. Patients reportedly had many misconceptions and fears about these tests and were embarrassed by having to remove their clothes for x-ray and other procedures. Nurses' observations during these examinations were also critical to the accurate interpretation of test results and, therefore, to accurate medical diagnosis. X-ray and laboratory work was deemed especially suited to the nurse who wanted to keep in touch with nursing, but who was less "adapted" by virtue of "physique or personality" to do continuous bedside nursing.[81] Nurses were, therefore, considered "natural(s)"[82] to assume the new work these tests generated as they were already serving in hospitals, had a great deal of knowledge about patients and diseases, and were already trained to be assistants to physicians.

Physician proponents of nurses in x-ray and laboratory fields, in particular, viewed nurses as especially suitable to assume the work of busy, absent, and unavailable physicians. Physicians could not have large caseloads of patients and the revenues they generated and also perform all the work the new diagnosis demanded. Accordingly, some of them turned to nurses as an available, cheap, and compliant alternative to house physicians. Lamenting the post–WWI shortage of interns in small hospitals, one North Carolina physician, Edmundson Boice, advocated the delegation of such "laborious" and "routine"[83] tasks as urinalysis, blood counts, and medical histories to nurses. Like other physicians, he had delegated these tasks to a "good nurse"[84] and was very satisfied with the results. According to Boice, a good nurse could assume more and more tasks until she was "almost as much assistance as a well trained house physician."[85] Arguably, by not having to compete for house physicians, hospitals risked lowering standards and losing the new ideas these physicians brought with them. Also, these house physicians could be paid less because this work would not be their life. A house physician worked for the experience, not the $25 per month he earned. In contrast, a nurse worked for what she earned, and she had to make laboratory work her life. However, according to Boice, delegating these tasks to nurses was ultimately the cheaper alternative since, once they were trained, there was no longer the cost of training a new house physician every year.

Although x-ray and laboratory work was promoted in the immediate post–WWI period and the 1920s as good for both nurses and physicians, nurses appear not to have entered these fields as specialists in numbers sufficient to meet the demand.[86] By the 1930s, advocates of nurse specialization promoted these fields to nurses for whom they were still "unknown land."[87] One physician reportedly lamented what he perceived as the timidity of most nurses who lacked the "ability and thirst for progression" that becoming a "roentgeonologist's assistant"[88] could satisfy. Nurses apparently still feared the dangers to health and fertility that x-ray work entailed. (Roentgenologists were reportedly initially reluctant to permit nurses near x-ray machines because of this danger.)[89] Moreover, this work was not always as interesting as advertised, typically involving routine and monotonous procedures. Also, this work was often simply added on to the nurse's ward work without any additional pay.[90] For all of its difficulties, most nurses likely preferred the intimacy of bedside care to the "science" of laboratory or x-ray work and did not see this work as essentially nursing work. Indeed, there is some indication that nurses saw x-ray and laboratory diagnosis as interfering with nursing work and the order of the ward.[91]

The "Over-Worked Eye"[92]

Especially after 1900, nurses acquired much of the labor of the new diagnosis. Instructional texts for nurses increasingly devoted more attention to the nurse's assistive role in medical diagnosis. By the 1930s, "assisting [the] physician in examining patients . . . and [in] making diagnostic tests" was one of twelve "aspects of nursing skill"[93] identified in a comprehensive activity analysis of nursing. In successive editions of the classic Harmer (and, later, Harmer and Virginia Henderson) textbooks on the principles and practice of nursing, what was topically referred to in 1922 as "nursing procedures"[94] used in the treatment of disease was, by 1939, described under the heading of "assisting with diagnostic procedures."[95] The Ewald Test Meal, for example, was a nursing procedure used to treat alimentary tract diseases in 1922, but in 1939 it was a diagnostic procedure that nurses assisted the physician to perform.

Physicians increasingly depended on nurses to detect and act on problems early as the nurse was likely to be the first one to discern an aberration in temperature or to find albumin in a patient's urine and, therefore, to spare the patient dangerous delays in treatment. Yet, although (or, perhaps, because) diagnosis was becoming a process to which nurses, patients, and others increasingly contributed, physicians sought to reserve the act of diagnosis exclusively for themselves. A recurring theme in instructional texts for nurses was that they were never to cross the line between nursing observation and medical diagnosis.[96] As one physician warned:

> Outside of correct reports, the nurse has nothing to do with diagnosis or prognosis. And, beyond executing orders and recording bedside notes, (she) has no part in the treatment.[97]

Nurses were repeatedly admonished in didactic texts that diagnosis was not their business, even as they were increasingly being offered and sought more scientific knowledge about disease and clinical experience in various components of diagnosis and as physicians were increasingly expecting nurses to perform de facto acts of diagnosis. Nurses were supposed to be able to distinguish between normal and abnormal conditions and to look for reasons for any abnormal findings. However, nurses were never to use the words normal or abnormal in reporting or recording patient conditions, and they were to refrain from offering their opinions on etiology or diagnosis.[98] Ethel Johns and Blanche Pfefferkorn summarized the paradoxical position of the nurse in relation to diagnosis by observing that:

> While the nurse is debarred from making a diagnosis, she is tacitly permitted to arrange into a pattern any significant symptoms upon which such diagnosis may be based.[99]

DIVIDING AND DENYING THE LABOR OF DIAGNOSIS

The new diagnostic technology reinforced the processual, as opposed to episodic, nature of diagnosis. This technology also both reinforced and blurred the line between the diagnosis that was supposed to be the physician's exclusive domain and the observation that was the nurse's shared domain.

A case in point involves the practice of clinical thermometry. When thermometers were first introduced into clinical practice, there seems to have been some concern among physicians about whether nurses or family members could be entrusted with their use. Physicians soon discovered, however, that the kind of information they needed for the diagnosis, treatment, and scientific study of disease required a graphic record of temperatures taken regularly and at critical moments in the progression of a disease, which, in turn, required someone at the bedside at the right times to obtain this information. Wunderlich, whose treatise was extremely influential in persuading physicians of the need for the thermometer in medical practice, contended that a major impediment to the practical utility of the thermometer was that it was too time-consuming for the physician to take all the temperatures he required.[100] Seguin had also noted that there was no part of the physician's work that required so much help as thermometry.[101] If only 1–2 temperature readings were needed, a physician could obtain these himself when he visited his patients. Indeed, if he could not, Seguin advised that the physician not take the case.[102] However, if 6–7 daily temperature readings were needed, the physician needed help; it was not necessary that he take the temperatures himself but only that he knew who took the temperatures and how they were taken. The physician's knowledge of pathological thermometry was sufficient to enable him to control or estimate the temperature readings obtained.

Moreover, anyone with good sight could be taught quickly to take accurate temperatures. Indeed, Wunderlich noted that persons unencumbered with the specialized knowledge of physicians were likely to make even fewer errors than the physician in obtaining an accurate temperature because they had no preconceived opinions to prejudice them.[103] In a similar vein, Seguin observed that

As astronomic observations are often better recorded by honest, attentive assistants than by astronomers, so a medical student, a nurse, (or) a relative can be made a useful assistant to the medical thermometrician.[104]

Yet, while Wunderlich noted the value and even necessity of assistants in performing the work of medical thermometry, he also believed that the "mere reading of temperature degrees helps diagnosis no more than dispensing does therapeusis."[105] Physicians minimized the skilled safety work involved in obtaining temperatures from children and delirious and fearful patients. Moreover, clinical thermometry was itself a technique that permitted the labor of diagnosis to be separated into unequal parts, with nurses increasingly assuming what were perceived as the largely mechanical tasks of taking and recording temperatures and of maintaining thermometers and physicians assuming what was perceived as the higher-order interpretive task of evaluating what the temperatures meant. By placing the tasks of diagnosis in a hierarchy and reserving the label of diagnosis only for physician acts of interpretation, physicians could deny that nonphysicians played any part in thermometric diagnosis, even as nurses were interpreting and expected to interpret temperature readings.

X-ray and laboratory technology also entailed an actual and rhetorical division and denial of labor. Nurses were seen as naturals to do much of the work of diagnosis without usurping the physician's preeminent role in diagnosis. Physicians in general practice were especially worried about the encroachment of x-ray and laboratory physician specialists (for example, pathologists and roentgenologists), who were competing for access to and revenues from patients by claiming the diagnostic act for themselves. Concerned over the abuse of medical specialization and overuse of the new diagnostic technologies, rank-and-file physicians were concerned that laboratories and x-ray units be seen as tools for the general physician—who knew the patient—to make diagnoses, not as diagnostic entities themselves.[106] Nurse specialization in these fields seemed neither to threaten physician access to patients nor, more importantly, their exclusive claim to diagnosis. The effect of this division and denial of the labor of diagnosis was to downplay the technical, interpersonal, and machine–body tending expertise of nurses and their frequently greater skill in these components of the application of the new technology to the patient.

EASY ENOUGH FOR A NURSE TO DO

The delegation to nurses of tasks considered easy enough for a nurse to do belied the actual complexity of these tasks. An especially good illustration of the complexity of tasks left to nurses was the Ewald Test Meal. This test was commonly used to diagnose gastrointestinal ailments and included a carefully sequenced and timed orchestration of events, which could involve up to four patients undergoing the test at the same time. According to Elizabeth Connolly, the superintendent of nursing at the North Carolina Sanatorium, 14 student nurses had successfully conducted 365 tests between 1921 and 1923. In her description of the procedure,[107] the test first involved patient preparation, which included instruction about the test and fasting. On the day of the test, with the patient resting in a recliner the nurse passed a rubber tube with a "bucket" (or tip designed to catch the gastric contents) into the stomach. This process often induced gagging in the patient, which the nurse reduced by spraying the throat with a 2% solution of cocaine. Once the tube was in the stomach, the nurse aspirated its contents with a syringe, taking care that the plunger not fit its barrel too snugly. Too tight a fit could cause the lining of the stomach to be damaged as it was sucked into the tip of the tube. The nurse then gave the patient the Ewald meal of bread and water, with or without the tube still in place. Removing it at this point meant that the nurse would have to reinsert it later rapidly enough to conform to the timing of events the test required. With a clock in full view the patient was given four minutes to finish the meal. If the nurse was supervising four patients at 2:45, this meant that patient 1 was required to finish the meal between 2:45 and 2:49; patient 2 was to finish between 2:49 and 2:53; patient 3 was to finish between 2:53 and 2:57; and patient 4 was to finish between 2:57 and 3:01. Exactly 11 minutes after the patient had finished the meal, the nurse aspirated the stomach contents. Patient 1 would have her or his stomach aspirated at 3:00, patient 2 would be aspirated at 3:04, patient 3 would be aspirated at 3:08, and patient 4 would be aspirated at 3:12. The nurse then placed the aspirated specimens into test tubes. She had to assure herself that the specimen was not bile-tinged, as that indicated that the bucket had passed out of the stomach into the duodenum, thereby invalidating the test. The nurse then removed the tube from the patient, taking care not to leave the bucket inside the stomach or esophagus and to avoid the laryngeal or pharyngeal spasms that often occurred during this process. Such spasms could greatly impede the tube's passage out of the patient. Tugging at the tube would both frighten the patient and further impede removal of the tube.

The "Over-Trained Nurse"

Assisting physicians with the new diagnosis required nurses to have new knowledge and skills in the application of devices and in enlisting patient cooperation for tests that could be uncomfortable, time-consuming, and/or frightening. However, even before technologically mediated diagnosis characterized medical practice, physicians were ambivalent about what nurses needed to know and, more important, should be taught to conduct the kind of close observation and reporting they required to prescribe treatment. On the one hand, many physicians saw nurses as Baconian data collectors, whose only frame of reference was to obtain the "raw data" the physician required. On the other hand, nurses were not just to report whatever they saw without interpretive comment but also to discern the likely reason for a symptom, to know what a symptom meant, and to take the required action.[108] Nurses were in the bizarre position of having to be mindful of symptoms without speaking their mind about them. Nurses were to "know . . . as much as the physician about the meaning of symptoms," yet they were to have no "tendency to become medical women, or to set up their own opinions in practice."[109]

Physicians' ambivalence about nurses' powers of observation and the education required to cultivate them is evident in the vigorous debate about the "overtrained nurse."[110] At times juxtaposed with the "under-trained"[111] physician the idea of the overtrained nurse emerged almost simultaneously with the actual appearance of trained nurses. A general concern of physicians who engaged in this debate was how much knowledge nurses should have for the good of patients and, perhaps, more important, for the good of physicians. Arguing that both a little and a lot of knowledge were dangerous to both patients and themselves, physicians were especially concerned that nurses not assume that either diagnosis or treatment was in their sphere.[112]

Especially troublesome to physicians most anxious about nursing education were examination questions for nurses that required answers only a physician should know and often did not.[113] As one physician argued, what patients required was not a nurse who could write a thesis about urinalysis or how to test for hydrochloric acid in stomach contents but, rather, one who could fluff their pillows, feed them, and report on their condition to the doctor. Indeed, advances in medical science and technology were causing both physicians and nurses to lose sight of the true and nonscientific function of the nurse.[114] As one physician summarized it:

> We do not want a scientific person; we do not want a person with theories of her own, or with a smattering of other people's theories . . . Of what use is it for [the nurse] . . . to hear lectures on the eye and the ophthalmoscope, subjects which occupy the earnest and constant study of highly educated men, and can be pursued to advantage by those only who give their whole time and attention to them?[115]

Conclusion: The Nurse's Eyes

Nurses played a central role in the technological transformation of medical practice and hospital care by putting the new diagnostic technology into use. Carl Mitcham differentiated between two views of technology as activity, that is, between activities that bring artifacts into existence and activities that put them to use.[116] Although nurses played no known part in the invention of the diagnostic devices addressd here, they did play a critical role in their application. Nurses performed key components of the work of medical diagnosis, variously obtaining device-mediated information from patients and recording, interpreting, and acting on this information. Nurses directly applied new devices and techniques to patients and they provided the before and after care of patients, and devices. The new "medical gaze" of the physician, accomplished with the aid of diagnostic technology, was, in part, "articulated through and mediated by" the nurse's eyes and hands.[117]

Yet, although nurses were essential to medical diagnosis, medical diagnosis was arguably not central to nursing. Instrumental diagnosis did not redefine nursing as it did medicine, where diagnosis replaced treatment in this period as the central point of the physician–patient encounter.[118] Nurses' encounters with patients around observation were still largely in-the-flesh; with the possible exception of the thermometer, there is little evidence that nurses used the information derived from these devices to alter nursing practice.[119] The new diagnostic technology seems to have altered the form more than the content of nursing work.

However, the new diagnostic technology complicated the work of the nurse and ideas about what nursing practice appropriately entailed. Nurses had more work to do in this realm, but whether this work drew nurses away from their traditional ministrations is still a matter for debate.[120] Perhaps less debatable—as it pertains to the development of modern American nursing— is that by blurring the dividing line between nursing observation and medical diagnosis, diagnostic technology was instrumental in both reinforcing and subverting the rhetorical and actual dividing line between nursing and doctoring. Clinical thermometry and x-ray and laboratory diagnosis, by their very material designs and the physical operations they entailed, reinforced the lines between medicine and nursing by permitting tasks to be divided into physical, mechanical, and interpretive components, which, in turn, could be delegated to nonphysicians or (at, the very least, rhetorically) reserved for physicians. Scopic techniques, by virtue of their not being so divisible (and, therefore, delegatable), also reinforced these lines.

These diagnostic techniques also subverted those lines by requiring the execution of tasks physicians often had insufficient time or skill to perform. While the delegation to nurses of tasks physicians considered easy enough for a nurse to do degraded the skill these tasks required, it also appears to have given nurses the opportunity to obtain more scientific knowledge and technical skill and to enter the new terrain of technological diagnosis. The diagnostic revolution required nurses to become skilled in tasks neither rhetorically nor legally delegated to them, as physicians expected nurses to stand in for them as doctors—that is, as diagnosticians—in their absence. By virtue of their absence and the constant presence of the nurse at the bedside, physicians had no choice but to depend on nurses, and nurses, in turn, had no choice—if patients were to be safe—but to perform de facto acts of diagnosis. Diagnostic technology did not create but rather illuminated the importance of this spatiotemporal asymmetry between medicine and nursing that favored nursing power.[121]

By making diagnosis central to medicine in this period the new technology also disempowered nursing. Before the diagnostic revolution in American medicine the focus of the physician–patient encounter was less on discerning the reason for an ailment than in alleviating its miseries. In the days prior to safe surgery and effective pharmacologic agents, medical treatment largely entailed good nursing care. With the new focus on diagnosis, even in the continuing absence of effective treatments for the diseases diagnosed, physicians gained power and control as the physician's diagnosis (obtaining it, confirming it, and/or being treated for it) was what brought patients into hospitals. In the new era of diagnosis, nursing seemed less autonomous and more dependent on medical diagnosis for its existence.

Accordingly, although nurses shared the use of many of the new diagnostic devices with physicians, they had different relations to them with different effects. Like the term technology itself, the nursing relation to the new diagnostic technology was "equivocal."[122] Nurses did not lose the close bonds they had with patients, which had arguably always been more intimate than physician–patient relations. They also did not gain the cultural authority that the new diagnostic technology conferred on physicians. Although they acquired new knowledge and skill, what nurses gained most of all was new (and, arguably, more) work to do. Diagnostic technology was also critical in elasticizing the sphere of the nurse; that is, this technology did not so much expand the sphere of influence of the nurse as permit her scope of responsibility to expand or contract according to whether physicians or others were available to perform the various tasks required by the technology. Whether a nurse did virtually all of the work associated with a diagnostic procedure or very little of it depended on the availability of other personnel and economic constraints. Yet, although the nurse's scope of responsibility was not fixed, there were certain duties that were relatively constant; nurses generally always cleaned up, and they always gained the cooperation of patients.

In an important sense the "doctor–nurse game" Leonard Stein described in 1967[123] began, in part, with the diagnostic revolution in medicine. However, it was then, as it remains even to this day, a game of words. Indeed, nurses would do well to understand language as practice and words as creators (as opposed to carriers) of meaning and reality. The denial of nonphysician diagnosis was largely a rhetorical move that became well entrenched in social custom, the law, and the popular imagination. The emergence of the nursing diagnosis movement in the 1960s was, in part, an effort to let physicians claim medical diagnosis while renaming and claiming the diagnostic work nurses actually performed.[124] The contemporary resurgence of the nurse practitioner has resurrected the debate about whether and what kind of diagnoses are in the nurse's proper sphere.

However, nurses promoting the nurse diagnostician with the argument that nursing and medical diagnoses are clearly defined and different entities would do well to consider the implications for nursing of the "conceptual acrobatics"[125] required to maintain this difference. Nurses promoting the nurse practitioner as the cheaper alternative to perform simple diagnostic acts would do well to remember that, in the history of nursing, skill has often appeared, not as an "objectively identifiable quality" but rather as an "ideological category" over which nurses have repeatedly been "denied the rights of contestation."[126]

MARGARETE SANDELOWSKI, PHD, RN, FAAN
PROFESSOR
DEPARTMENT OF WOMEN'S AND CHILDREN'S HEALTH
UNIVERSITY OF NORTH CAROLINA AT CHAPEL HILL
SCHOOL OF NURSING
7460 CARRINGTON HALL
CHAPEL HILL, NC 27599

Notes

1. Robert A. Kilduffe, "The Nurse and Her Relation to Symptomatology, I: The Pulse," *Trained Nurse and Hospital Review* 65, no. 6 (1920): 498.

2. Rosemary Stevens, *In Sickness and in Wealth: American Hospitals in the Twentieth Century* (New York: Basic Books, 1989). According to Stevens (p. 12), nurses were "captured by the hospital and institutionally subsumed."

3. Anselm Strauss et al., "Sentimental Work in the Technologized Hospital," *Sociology of Health & Illness* 4, no. 3 (1982): 254–77.

4. The classic work in this field is Stanley Joel Reiser, *Medicine and the Reign of Technology* (Cambridge, U.K.: Cambridge University Press, 1978). See also by Reiser, "Technology and the Eclipse of Individualism in Medicine," *The Pharos* 45, no. 1 (1982): 10–15; "The Science of Diagnosis: Diagnostic Technology," in *Companion Encyclopedia of the History of Medicine*, ed. W. F. Bynum and Roy Porter (London: Routledge, 1993), 2:826–51; and, "Technology and the Use of the Senses in Twentieth-Century Medicine," in *Medicine and the Five Senses*, eds. W. F. Bynum and Roy Porter (Cambridge, U.K.: Cambridge University Press, 1993), 262–73. Other key

scholarship in this field includes the works of Joel D. Howell and Audrey B. Davis. See Howell's "Early Use of X-ray Machines and Electrocardiographs at the Pennsylvania Hospital, 1897 through 1927," *Journal of the American Medical Association* 255, no. 17 (1986): 2320–23; *Technology and American Medical Practice. 1880–1930: Anthology of Sources* (New York: Garland Press, 1988); "Machines and Medicine: Technology Transforms the American Hospital," in *The American General Hospital: Communities and Social Contexts,* ed. Diana Elizabeth Long and Janet Golden (Ithaca, N.Y.: Cornell University Press, 1989), 109–34; and, *Technology in the Hospital: Transforming Patient Care in the Early Twentieth Century* (Baltimore: Johns Hopkins University Press, 1995). See Davis, *Medicine and its Technology: An Introduction to the History of Medical Instrumentation* (Westport, Conn.: Greenwood Press, 1981); and "American Medicine in the Gilded Age: The First Technological Era," *Annals of Science* 47 (1990): 111–25.

5. For the growing importance of "science" in this period, the association of new diagnostic instrumentation with science, and physicians' effective use of the rhetoric of science, see Merriley Borell, "Training the Senses, Training the Mind," in *Medicine and the Five Senses,* ed. W. F. Bynum and Roy Porter (Cambridge, U.K.: Cambridge University Press, 1993), 244–61; Charles E. Rosenberg, *No Other Gods: On Science and American Social Thought,* rev. ed. (Baltimore: Johns Hopkins University Press, 1997); S. E. D. Shortt, "Physicians, Science, and Status: Issues in the Professionalization of Anglo-American Medicine in the Nineteenth Century," *Medical History* 27 (1983): 51–68; and, Ronald G. Walters, ed., *Scientific Authority and Twentieth-Century America* (Baltimore: Johns Hopkins University Press, 1997).

6. Hughes Evans, "Losing Touch: The Controversy Over the Introduction of Blood Pressure Instruments into Medicine," *Technology and Culture* 34, no. 4 (1993): 784–807.

7. Evans, "Losing Touch," 799.

8. Reiser, "Technology and the Eclipse of Individualism," 12.

9. Reiser, "Science of Diagnosis," 829.

10. Bertha Harmer, *Textbook of the Principles and Practice of Nursing* (New York: Macmillan, 1922), 45.

11. See, for example, Patricia Benner, ed., *Interpretive Phenomenology: Embodiment, Caring, and Ethics in Health and Illness* (Thousand Oaks, Calif.: Sage, 1994); Donald A. Laird, *Applied Psychology for Nurses* (Philadelphia: J. B. Lippincott, 1923); Hildegard E. Peplau, *Interpersonal Relations in Nursing* (New York: G.P. Putnam's Son, 1952); and, Christine A. Tanner et al., "The Phenomenology of Knowing the Patient," *Image: Journal of Nursing Scholarship* 25, no. 4 (1993): 273–80.

12. David Armstrong, "The Fabrication of Nurse–Patient Relationships, *Social Science & Medicine* 17, no. 8 (1983): 457–60.

13. Florence Nightingale, *Notes on Nursing: What It Is and What It Is Not* (New York: Dover, 1969/1860), 105.

14. Nightingale, *Notes,* 106.

15. Nightingale, *Notes,* 106.

16. Nightingale, *Notes,* 109.

17. Charles E. Rosenberg, *The Care of Strangers: The Rise of America's Hospital System* (Baltimore: Johns Hopkins University Press, 1987); and John H. Warner, *The*

The Therapeutic Perspective: Medical Practice. Knowledge, and Identity in America. 1820–1885 (Cambridge, Mass.: Harvard University Press, 1986).

18. Nightingale, *Notes,* 133.

19. Nightingale, Notes, 110.

20. Nightingale, *Notes,* 111.

21. Nightingale, *Notes,* 116.

22. Nightingale, *Notes,* 124.

23. See, for example, Bellevue Hospital, *A Manual of Nursing* (New York: G. P. Putnam's Sons, 1878), 23–35; Harmer, *Textbook,* 45–49; Isabel Hampton Robb, *Nursing: Its Principles and Practice for Hospital and Private Use,* 3rd ed. (Cleveland, Ohio: E. C. Koeckert, 1906), 253–69.

24. Philadelphia General Hospital, *Nursing Procedures,* 1924, Center for the Study of the History of Nursing, University of Pennsylvania, School of Nursing, p. 120 (hereafter cited as CSHN).

25. Clara S. Weeks, *A Textbook of Nursing* (New York: D. Appleton, 1890), 80.

26. Weeks, *Textbook,* 80

27. Robb, *Nursing,* 41.

28. See, for example, the following series written by a physician: Robert A. Kilduffe, "The Nurse and Her Relation to Symptomatology, I: The Pulse," *Trained Nurse and Hospital Review,* 65, no. 6 (1920): 498–501 (hereafter cited to as TNHR); "The Nurse and Her Relation to Symptomatology, II: The Temperature," TNHR 66, no. 1 (1921): 13–16; and "The Nurse and Her Relation to Symptomatology, III: The Respiration," TNHR 66, no. 2 (1921): 109–12.

29. See, for example, the series by Myer Solis-Cohen, "How to Observe Symptoms," TNHR 35 (July 1905): 8–11, (August 1905): 83–85, and (September 1905): 140–42; and, Eugene A. Smith, "The Observation of Symptoms," *Trained Nurse* 1, no. 1 (1888): 52–55.

30. See, for example, Weeks, *Textbook,* 80.

31. Log, 26 August 1888, Mary U. Clymer Papers, CSHN.

32. Agnes B. Meade, "Training the Senses in Clinical Observation," TNHR 97, no. 6 (1936): 540–44. Quote on p. 540.

33. John D. Thompson and Grace Goldin, *The Hospital: A Social and Architectural History* (New Haven, Conn.: Yale University Press, 1975), 232. "Supervision/ observability" (p. 231) competed with "privacy" (p. 207) in the history of hospital design. That is, as more patients were housed in private rooms, nurses found it harder to maintain visual control of patients and the environment surrounding them. With the increasing replacement of the ward with the private room a nurse could no longer stand at one point in a ward and see everything she needed to see.

34. In Linda Richards, *Reminiscenses of Linda Richards: America's First Trained Nurse* (Boston, Mass.: Whitcomb & Barrows, 1911), 18–19, Richards suggested an important early environmental impediment to nursing observation. Concerning night duty at Bellevue Hospital, she recalled:

> No sooner had the day nurses left the wards than the gas was turned so low that the faces of the patients could not be distinguished. One could only see the dim outlines of figures wrapped in gray blankets lying upon the beds. If any work

was to be done, a candle must be lighted, and only two candles a week were allowed each ward. If more were used, the nurse had to provide them . . . The captain of the watch . . . at 5 A.M. . . . turned off all the gas, leaving us in total darkness. Richards had this practice reversed by promising that nurses would use no more gas than they required to fulfill their duties.

35. See, for example, Borell, "Training the Senses"; Malcolm Nicolson, "The Art of Diagnosis: Medicine and the Five Senses," in *Companion Encyclopedia of the History of Medicine*, eds. W. F. Bynum and Roy Porter (London: Routledge, 1993), 2:801–25; and, Reiser, "Science of Diagnosis."

36. S. Weir Mitchell, *The Early History of Instrumental Precision in Medicine*, (New Haven, Conn.: Tuttle, Morehouse, and Taylor, 1892).

37. Martha E. Erdmann and Margaret Welsh, "Studies in Thermometer Technique," *Nursing Education Bulletin* 2, no. 1 (1929): 8–33. Quote on p. 11. See also, on the history of clinical thermometry, Logan Clendening, "The History of Certain Medical Instruments," *Annals of Internal Medicine* 4, no. 2 (1930): 176–89; J. Gershon-Cohen, "A Short History of Medical Thermometry," *Annals of the New York Academy of Sciences* 121 (1964): 4–11; Hugh A. McGuigan, "Medical Thermometry," *Annals of Medical History* 9, no. 2 (1937): 148–54; and Reiser, *Medicine and the Reign of Technology*, 91–121.

38. Carl A. Wunderlich, *On the Temperature in Diseases: A Manual of Medical Thermometry*, trans. W. Bathurst Woodman (London: New Sydenham Society, 1871).

39. Edouard Seguin, *Family Thermometry: A Manual of Thermometry for Mothers, Nurses, Hospitalers, Etc., and All Those Who Have Charge of the Sick and the Young* (New York: Putnam, 1873); and *Medical Thermometry and Human Temperature*, 2nd ed. (New York: William Wood, 1876). Excerpts of Sequin, *Family Thermometry* are reprinted in *Temperature, Part 1: Arts and Concepts*, ed. Theodore H. Benzinger (Stroudsburg, Pa.: Dowden, Hutchinson & Ross, 1977), 316–335.

40. Seguin, *Medical Thermometry*, 253.

41. See, for example, Amanda Beck, *A Reference Handbook for Nurses* (Philadelphia: W. B. Saunders, 1905), 50; Harmer, *Textbook*, 134–151; and Lecture 21 November 1887, Mary U. Clymer Papers, CSHN.

42. See the ads at the back of Bellevue Hospital, *Manual of Nursing*, and Emily M. A. Stoney, *Bacteriology and Surgical Technique for Nurses* (Philadelphia: W. B. Saunders, 1900).

43. See, for example, Frank S. Betz Company, *Surgical Instruments and Supplies*, 1918, Medical Trade Ephemera Collection, College of Physicians of Philadelphia, p. 37; Anna M. Fullerton, *Surgical Nursing* (Philadelphia: P. Blakiston's Son, 1899), 255; E. Hibbard, "A Nurse's Requirements," *Trained Nurse* 2, no. 5 (1889): 188–89; Emily A. M. Stoney, *Practical Points in Nursing for Nurses in Private Practice*, 2nd ed. (Philadelphia: W. B. Saunders, 1897), 25; and, H. W. Weed Company, *Illustrations of Surgical Instruments*, 1902, Medical Trade Catalog Collection, Division of Medical Sciences, National Museum of American History, Washington, D.C., p. 2115.

44. See the Becton, Dickinson ad located before the table of contents, *American Journal of Nursing* 27 (April 1927).

45. See, for example, Alice Ward Bailey, "Hospital Life," *Scribner's Magazine* 3 (1888): 698–715; Emily Bax, "Are Nurses Overpaid?" *Hygeia* 9 (1931, August):

727–31, quote on p. 727; Katherine DeWitt, "Hospital Sketches," *American Journal of Nursing* 6, no. 7 (1906): 455–59.

    46. Isabel A. Hampton, *Nursing: Its Principles and Practice* (Philadelphia: W. B. Saunders, 1893), 93.

    47. Seguin, *Family Thermometry*, 4.

    48. Seguin, *Family Thermometry*, 5.

    49. Seguin, *Family Thermometry*, 19.

    50. Seguin, *Family Thermometry*, 19–20.

    51. Seguin, *Family Thermometry*, 20.

    52. Bellevue Hospital, *Manual of Nursing*, 143.

    53. Connecticut Training School for Nurses, *A Handbook of Nursing for Family and General Use* (Philadelphia: J. B. Lippincott, 1879), 107–9.

    54. Hampton, *Nursing*, 167–85.

    55. Hampton, *Nursing*, 170.

    56. Hampton, *Nursing*, 184.

    57. J. C. Wilson, *Fever Nursing* (Philadelphia: J. B. Lippincott, 1899).

    58. Harmer, *Textbook*, 138.

    59. Helen W. Faddis et al., "Making Temperature Taking Safe," *Pacific Coast Journal of Nursing* 24, no. 2 (1928): 73–74.

    60. A contemporary concept with historical relevance described by Shizuko Fagerhaugh et al., "Chronic Illness, Medical Technology, and Clinical Safety in the Hospital," *Research in the Sociology of Health Care* 4 (1986): 237–70.

    61. See, for example, the Becton, Dickinson ad, TNHR 66, no. 1 (1921): 73; the Faichney Instrument ad, *Hospital Management* 21, no. 2 (1926): 88; and Minnie Goodnow, *The Technic of Nursing* (Philadelphia: W. B. Saunders, 1928), 148.

    62. Daisy Barnwell Jones, *My First Eighty Years* (Baltimore: Gateway Press, 1986), 250. A student at Johns Hopkins in the late 1920s and early 1930s, she described having fallen and, as a result, broken 32 thermometers for which she did not have to pay. This book is available at the North Carolina Collection (hereafter referred to as NCC), University of North Carolina at Chapel Hill, N.C.

    63. Erdmann and Walsh, "Studies in Thermometer Technique," 8–33. See also Ruth Ashburn, "A Bacteriological Study of Clinical Thermometer Technic," *American Journal of Nursing* 30, no. 3 (1930): 336–42 (hereafter cited as AJN); A. Frances Fischer and Catherine Simonds, "A Modern Hospital Takes its Temperatures," AJN 29, no. 1 (1929): 89–90;

    64. See, for example, Goodnow, *Technic*, 148; Harmer, *Textbook*, 150; and Weeks, *Textbook*, 67.

    65. Hampton, *Nursing*, 50.

    66. See, for example, Faddis et al., "Making Temperature Taking Safe," 74; Harriet M. Gillette, "A Practical Thermometer Tray," AJN 26, no. 11 (1926): 840; and "A Method of Taking Temperatures," AJN 27, no. 10 (1927): 810.

    67. See, for example, Minnie Goodnow, *First-Year Nursing: A Textbook for Pupils During Their First Year of Hospital Work*, 2nd ed. (Philadelphia: W. B. Saunders, 1919), 138.

    68. See, for example, Joseph B. Cooke, *A Nurse's Handbook of Obstetrics*, 10th ed. (Philadelphia: J. B. Lippincott, 1924); Joseph B. DeLee, *Obstetrics for Nurses*, 9th eds.

(1913; reprint, Philadelphia: W. B. Saunders, 1930); and Carolyn Conant Van Blarcom, *Obstetrical Nursing*, 3rd eds. (1922; reprint, New York: Macmillan, 1922 and 1933).

69. See, for example, Robert A. Kilduffe, "The Blood Pressure: A Consideration of Its Technique and Significance," TNHR 68 (March, 1922): 228–30; Louise Gliem, "High Blood Pressure: Its Care and Treatment," AJN 24, no. 12 (1924): 1184–89; Veronica F. Murray ("Technic of Taking Blood Pressure," AJN 34, no. 11 (1934): 1057–64; Charles C. Sutter, "Blood Pressure," AJN 15, no. 1 (1915): 7–13; William S. Middleton, "Blood Pressure Determination: A Nursing Procedure," AJN 30, no. 10 (1930): 1219–25; and Irving Wilson Voorhies, "What Is Blood Pressure?" TNHR 61 (1918, July) 6–8. The Philadelphia General Hospital School of Nursing did not include the taking of blood pressure in its procedure books until 1948. See Philadelphia General Hospital, *Nursing Procedures*, 40. In DeLee's *Obstetrics for Nurses*, p. 116, a nurse is shown taking the blood pressure. Blood pressure technique is not described at all in, for example, Barbara A. Thompson, *Nursing Procedures: A manual Used in the Teaching of the Principles and Practice of Nursing in the Associated Hospitals in the University of Minnesota School of Nursing* (Minneapolis: The University of Minnesota Press, 1929; and Mary C. Wheeler and Arnalia Metzker, *Nursing Technic* (Philadelphia: J. B. Lippincott, 1930).

70. Evans, "Losing Touch," 784–807.

71. Smith, "The Observation of Symptoms," 53.

72. For more on media images of nurses and physicians, see, for example, Daniel M. Fox and Christopher Lawrence, *Photographing Medicine: Images and Power in Britain and America Since 1840* (New York: Greenwood Press, 1988); and N. J. Krantzler, "Media Images of Physicians and Nurses in the United States," *Social Science & Medicine* 22 (1986): 933–52.

73. See, for example, Howell, *Technology in the Hospital*; Reiser, *Medicine and the Reign of Technology*; and Stanley J. Reiser, "The Test Tube As Oracle: The Domination of Diagnostics by Laboratory Analysis," in *History of Diagnostics*, ed. Yosio Kawakita (Proceedings of the 9th International Symposium on the Comparative History of Medicine—East and West, (Osaka, Japan: The Taniguchi Foundation, 1987), 175–85.

74. See, for example, Stevens, *In Sickness and in Wealth*, 105–31.

75. See, for example, P. C. Remondino, "The Trained Nurse in Private Practice," *Trained Nurse* 32, no. 2 (1904): 77–82; and Weeks, *Textbook*, 173.

76. See, for example, Annual Report of the Watts Hospital for the Year Ending 30 November 1922, NCC, Durham, NC., p. 41; and "Suggestions for National Hospital Day Publicity," *Bulletin of the American Hospital Association* 1, no. 1 (1927): 3–23.

77. For the varied duties and education of the nurse in these fields, see, for example, Charlotte A. Aikens, *Clinical Studies for Nurses*, 2nd ed. (Philadelphia: W. B. Saunders, 1912), 37; Sister Alma, *Clinical Laboratory Manual for Nurses and Technicians* (St. Louis: C. V. Mosby, 1932); Louise B. D'Arby, "The Hospital X-ray Nurse," AJN 17, no. 6 (1917): 488–90; Louise B. D'Arby, "Suggestions for the X-ray Room, II: Fluoroscopic Work and Record Keeping," TNHR 70, no. 5 (1923):

416–17; Henry J. Goeckel, "A Plan for the Laboratory Training of Nurses," *Modern Hospital* 12 (1919, June): 422–23; A. Hazelwood, "The Nurse and the Clinical Laboratory," AJN 27, no. 4 (1927): 259–61; R. M. L. "My Experience in X-ray Work," AJN 20, no. 8 (1920): 626–27; Rose M. Lorish, "The Development of the X-ray Negative," AJN 21, no. 4 (1921): 234–36; Margaret Ossenback, "Training School for Nurses," in the Annual Report of the Watts Hospital for the Year Ending 30 November 1921, NCC, Durham, N.C., pp. 22–27; Olive B. Sweet, "A Hospital Nurse's Day," *U. S. Veterans' Bureau Medical Bulletin* 1, no. 4 (1925): 57–61; Catherine B. Washburn, "Assisting With Diagnostic Tests," AJN 29, no. 6 (1929): 645–48; Edith L. Weart, "The Nurse as Laboratory Technician," AJN 32, no. 12 (1912): 1251–54; and, John B. Zingrone, "Mercy Hospital X-ray Laboratory," *Hospital Progress* 1, no. 3 (1920): 104–7. See also the series by Henry J. Goeckel, "The Laboratory: Its Relation to the Nursing Service," TNHR 70, nos. 1– 6 (1923): 44–45, 115–16, 226–27, 320–21, 413–15, and 509–11.

78. See, for example, Nora D. Dean, "The Roentgenological Field for Nurses," AJN 21, no. 3 (1920): 159–61; E. Blanche Seyfert, "Opportunities for the Nurse in the X-ray Diagnostic Laboratory," TNHR 68 (February 1922): 136–37. Quote on p. 136.

79. J. M. Parrott, response to Edmundson S. Boice, "The Interne Problem of the Small Hospital," Transactions of the North Carolina Hospital Association, NCC, Pinehurst, N.C., pp. 14–19, quote on p. 19.

80. See, for example, Seyfert, "Opportunities for the Nurse"; M. Warwick "The Nurse As Laboratory Technician," AJN 27, no. 2 (1927): 95–97; and, Weart, "Nurse as Laboratory Technician."

81. Seyfert, "Opportunities for the Nurse," 137.

82. Seyfert, "Opportunities for the Nurse," 137.

83. Boice, "Interne Problem," 18.

84. Boice, "Interne Problem," 18.

85. Boice, "Interne Problem," 18.

86. I have as yet found no means to determine exactly how many nurses assumed these roles. A nurse is listed as a laboratory technician in the Annual Report of the Watts Hospital for the Year Ending 30 November 1921, NCC, Durham, N.C., p. 7.

87. Weart, "Nurse as Laboratory Technician," 1251.

88. Seyfert, "Opportunities for the Nurse," 137.

89. D'Arby, "Hospital X-ray Nurse," 488; Dean, "Roentgenological Field," 159; and Seyfert, "Opportunities for the Nurse," 138.

90. Warwick, "Nurse as Laboratory Technician," 97.

91. Mabel McVicker, "The Importance of Understanding Medical Laboratory Tests," AJN 23, no. 1 (1922): 14–16. On p. 14, McVicker wrote that too often, nurses looked on a "test" as something that had to be done because a doctor ordered it and felt relief when it was over because the "routine" work of the ward could then proceed without further interference. However, according to McVicker, nurses would do this work with interest, enthusiasm, and accuracy if they knew the significance of the test and the importance of nurses in assisting with diagnosis.

92. Maud Banfield, "The Cleaning," in *On the Administrative Frontier of Medicine: The First Ten Years of the American Hospital Association. 1899–1908*, ed.

Morris J. Vogel (New York: Garland, 1989), 59–62. On p. 61, she uses this phrase in a different context to refer to the superintendent of nurses who tries to "keep an eye" on cleaning.

93. Ethel Johns and Blanche Pfefferkorn, *An Activity Analysis of Nursing* (New York: Committee on the Grading of Nursing Schools, 1934), 83.

94. Harmer, *Textbook,* xi.

95. Bertha Harmer and Virginia Henderson, *Textbook of the Principles and Practice of Nursing,* 4th ed. (New York: Macmillan, 1939), ix.

96. See, for example, Charlotte A. Aikens, *Studies in Ethics for Nurses* (Philadelphia: W. B. Saunders, 1916), 112–13; George H. Hoxie, *Practice of Medicine for Nurses: A Textbook for Nurses and Students of Domestic Science, and a Handbook for All Those Who Care for the Sick* (Philadelphia: W. B. Saunders, 1980), preface; Kilduffe, "The Nurse and Her Relation to Symptomatology," 498.

97. Smith, "The Observation of Symptoms," 54.

98. See, for example, Goodnow, *First-Year Nursing,* 197; and Solis-Cohen, "How to Observe Symptoms," 8.

99. Johns and Pfefferkorn, *Activity Analysis,* 21.

100. Wunderlich, *On the Temperature in Diseases,* 74.

101. Seguin, *Medical Thermometry,* 281.

102. Seguin, *Medical Thermometry,* 281.

103. Wunderlich, *On the Temperature in Diseases,* 75.

104. Seguin, *Medical Thermometry,* 281.

105. Wunderlich, *On the Temperature in Diseases,* 75.

106. Reiser, "Test Tube as Oracle," and "Technology and the Eclipse of Individualism." On the use and abuse of laboratory diagnosis (with an emphasis on the debate in North Carolina), see also, for example, Richard C. Cabot, "The Historical Development and Relative Value of Laboratory and Clinical Methods of Diagnosis," *Boston Medical and Surgical Journal* 157, no. 5 (1907): 150–53 (hereafter referred to as BMSJ); Robert H. Lafferty, "The Importance of Chemistry and Physiology to the General Practitioner," *Transactions of the Medical Society of the State of North Carolina* 59 (1912): 498–501 (hereafter referred to as TMSNC); Paul H. Ringer, "Abuse of the Laboratory From the Viewpoint of the Laboratory Worker," TMSNC 57 (1910): 377–81; John H. Tucker, "What Aid is the Laboratory in Diagnosis?" TMSNC 58 (1911): 532–36; S. A. Stevens, "The Relation of the Specialist to the General Practitioner," TMSNC 58 (1911): 172–77; W. H. Prioleau, "What Laboratory Work Should Be Done By The Physician Himself?" TMSNC 51 (1904): 324–27.

107. Elizabeth Connolly, "The Nurse and the Fractional Ewald Meal by the Rehfus Method," in Transactions of the Sixth Annual Meeting of the North Carolina Hospital Association, NCC, Asheville, N.C., pp. 80–84.

108. See, for example, J. M. Davis, "Teaching Bacteriology in School [sic] of Nursing," in Official Proceedings of the 32nd Annual Convention of the North Carolina State Nurses' Association, 25–27 October 1934, NCC, Fayetteville, N.C., pp. 59–63; Kilduffe, "The Nurse and Her Relation to Symptomatology"; Smith, "The Observation of Symptoms"; Solis Cohen, "How to Observe Symptoms."

109. Dr. Billings quoted in Ethel Johns and Blanche Pfefferkorn, *The Johns Hopkins Hospital School of Nursing, 1889–1949* (Baltimore: Johns Hopkins Press, 1954), 13.

110. See, for example, W. Gilman Thompson, "The Overtrained Nurse," *New York Medical Journal* 83, no. 17 (1906): 845–49.

111. Thompson, "Overtrained Nurse," 846.

112. See, for example, Richard O. Beard, "The Education of the Nurse in America," *Transactions of the American Hospital Association* 12 (1910): 345–59; Richard C. Cabot, "Suggestions for the Improvement of Training Schools for Nurses," BMSJ 145, no. 21 (1901): 567–69; Thelma Ingles, "The Physicians' View of the Evolving Nursing Profession," *Nursing Forum* 15, no. 2 (1976): 123–64; and "Nursing as a Profession," BMSJ 149, no. 5 (1903): 133–34; John H. Packard, "On the Training of Nurses for the Sick," BMSJ XCV, no. 20 (1876): 573–79; and "The Reciprocal Relations of the Nurse and the Physician," BMSJ 121, no. 17 (1889): 417–18; G. H. M. Rowe, "The Training of Nurses," BMSJ 109, no. 1 (1883): 1–4.

113. See, for example, President's Address, in Transactions of the North Carolina Hospital Association, 20 April 1920, NCC, Charlotte, N.C., p. 8. A physician is quoted as saying: "Don't make a poor doctor and spoil a good nurse."

114. Thompson, "Overtrained Nurse," 848.

115. Packard, "On the Training of Nurses," 577.

116. Carl Mitcham, *Thinking Through Technology: The Path Between Engineering and Philosophy* (Chicago: University of Chicago Press, 1994), 209. What is often forgotten is that most physicians also did not bring technologies into existence but, rather, put them to use. We tend to valorize invention over application and to see physicians (males) as inventors and nurses (females) as only users.

117. Eva Gamarnikow, "Nurse or Woman: Gender and Professionalism in Reformed Nursing, 1860–1923," in *Anthropology and Nursing*, eds. Pat Holden and Jenny Littlewood (London: Routledge, 1986), 110–29. Quote on p. 119. Gamarnikow studied British nursing.

118. Toby Gelfand, "The History of the Medical Profession," in *Companion Encyclopedia*, 1119–50.

119. The lack of evidence here may be more a consequence of the serious lack of data available to researchers concerning actual nursing practice than a reflection of nurses' nonuse of such technological information as the results of x-ray and laboratory tests. Yet, even textbooks of the period emphasize the nurses' role in acquiring the information for physicians as opposed to using the information themselves in nursing practice.

120. Blanche Pfefferkorn and Marian Rottman, *Clinical Education in Nursing* (New York: Macmillan, 1932). In the section "Extra-Nursing Functions and the Nursing Load," 51–52, these nurses noted that:

> An idea frequently expressed is that technical and medical functions are being steadily transferred to the nursing staff, with encroachment on nursing duties and greatly increased nursing load. This may be true in so far as graduate nurses elect work of that type. Findings from the Bellevue Study reveal an almost negligible amount of time given to activities, other than those of a purely nursing nature. . . . If the assignment, taking and recording of blood pressure, to the nursing staff, adds two hours to a daily load of 100 hours, the increase is not sufficient to burden the nursing service or to affect the quality of the nursing. It seems likely that the time emphasis placed upon new responsibilities outside the immediate field of nursing has been due to the fact that in most

institutions, the required nursing load hours exceed the provided nursing hours, and, as a result, any addition to the already existing load is apt to be considered out of its right proportion.

121. Davina Allen, "The Nursing–Medical Boundary: A Negotiated Order?" *Sociology of Health & Illness* 19, no. 4 (1997): 498–520.

122. Mitcham, *Thinking Through Technology*, 152.

123. Leonard Stein, "The Doctor–Nurse Game," *Archives of General Psychiatry* 16 (June 1967): 699–703.

124. Marjory Gordon, *Nursing Diagnosis: Process and Application*, 3rd ed. (St. Louis, Mo.: Mosby, 1994).

125. Gamarnikow, "Nurse or Woman," 123.

126. Rosalind Gill and Keith Grint, "The Gender-Technology Relation: Contemporary Theory and Research," in *The Gender-Technology Relation: Contemporary Theory and Research*, ed. Keith Grint and Rosalind Gill (London: Taylor & Francis, 1995), 1–28. Quote on p. 9.

Eleanor Clarke Slagle and Susan E. Tracy:
Personal and Professional Identity and the Development of Occupational Therapy in Progressive Era America

VIRGINIA A. METAXAS

Department of History
Southern Connecticut State University

In March of 1917 the National Society for the Promotion of Occupational Therapy[1] held its organizational meeting in Clifton Springs, New York. Eleanor Clarke Slagle, a mental hygiene activist from Hull House, Chicago, and Susan E. Tracy, a Massachusetts nurse and well-respected author of occupational therapy's first textbook *Studies in Invalid Occupation* (1910), were two of the founders who sought to move occupational therapy from its origins in reform to what Dr. Herbert J. Hall called "a new profession for women." In seeking a unified vision for the field the founding generation took principles and practices from nursing, teaching, medicine, psychiatry, arts and crafts, rehabilitation, self-help, orthopedics, mental hygiene, social work, and more to enrich the depth and breadth of occupational therapy's professional panorama.

Yet, drawing from these varied perspectives caused problems. Because the first generation of occupational therapists came from various professional fields or, more accurately, from several professions-in-the-making, they found it difficult to create a concise body of knowledge, authority, and identity in the early 20th century's evolving culture of professionalism and medical hierarchy.[2] In a time when scientific medicine seemed to be nearly obsessed with measurement—what healthcare professionals might today call "patient outcomes"—occupational therapists struggled to determine objective criteria by which to assess occupational therapy's value. The dilemmas of balancing the scientific and humanistic trends inherent in occupational therapy, of finding occupational therapy's place in American medicine, and of meeting the aims

Nursing History Review 8 (2000): 39-70. A publication of the American Association for the History of Nursing.

of scientific medicine shaped the agenda of the first generation of occupational therapists during the 1910s and 1920s.

An important strategy used by the leaders of occupational therapy to legitimize the new female-dominated profession in the world of medicine and in the general public was to draw upon the dual authority of male physicians (within their ranks) and female charity networks. Male and female founders instituted a gender-defined division of labor in building the profession.[3] The men, essentially, built the necessary bridges between occupational therapy and the largely male medical world. They instituted the expected trappings of a profession, such as developing a theoretical base and publishing a journal with research findings. Furthermore, the men took positions of authority in the American Occupational Therapy Association. From its founding in 1917 until after the World War II (with the exception of one year), male physicians or men closely related to mainstream medicine served as presidents of the association. Often, as well, physicians held conspicuous positions on boards of training schools and practice clinics as another strategy toward legitimizing occupational therapy in the medical world.

However, I do not see this as a male attempt to take over the profession, and surely, I do not mean to say that women played passive roles in building the profession. Women within and outside of the profession actively forged this female-dominated healthcare profession. For example, most schools and clinics that trained and provided workplaces for occupational therapists since 1917 were founded, underwritten, and managed by a cooperating community of women practitioners and charity women, often members of women's clubs or charity groups such as the Junior League or the Red Cross. As a result, these institutions held a generous degree of autonomy and freedom from male-dominated medical and educational institutions, resting instead upon a rich tradition of 19th-century American women's volunteer and charity activities.

Occupational therapists, though, were not completely comfortable with drawing upon 19th-century traditions of working closely with charity women. They, like many other aspiring women professionals of the Progressive Era, often found themselves caught between traditional and modern female roles. They were not satisfied with identifying themselves as volunteer altruists, nor did they necessarily wish to internalize male models of professionalism. Their story is one of walking a tightrope between two worlds—those of medicine and women's reform.

In this article I will focus on two tensions characteristic of this newly emerging predominantly female profession: (1) the personal identity of the founding women and (2) the ways that two women of the founding generation juggled competing influences from neighboring professions such as social work, mental hygiene, education, and nursing in order to create new professional boundaries for occupational therapy. I will examine the careers of Eleanor Clarke Slagle and Susan E. Tracy because they were perceived to be leaders of the first generation of occupational therapy and because their respective visions of occupational therapy differed substantially, as did their personal identities. Slagle sought independence for occupational therapy; her ambition was to see it as an autonomous medical specialty. Slagle helped organize the founding of the profession's first national organization in 1917, and she welcomed the cooperation of medical men such as psychiatrists William Rush Dunton Jr., Hall, and Adolph Meyer. Slagle held highly visible and powerful leadership roles in the profession until her retirement in 1937—indeed, she was so admired by her contemporaries that they designated her "the Jane Addams of occupational therapy." Tracy, like Slagle, made important contributions to the founding of occupational therapy as a field and likewise was held in great esteem by her contemporaries. Unlike Slagle, Tracy did not actively participate in *professionalizing* occupational therapy because she wanted it to be a subspecialty of nursing. She believed that occupational therapy could serve as a tool for nurses in their work with convalescing patients. Less comfortable than Slagle with interacting with the male medical establishment and struggling with national issues surrounding the evolving profession, Tracy instead focused on building local institutions and training newcomers to the field. After a few short years of work in the occupational therapy movement, Tracy returned to nursing, the profession with which she primarily identified, where she remained active until her death in 1927.

The Context: Medicine and Women's Reform

When occupational therapy first appeared in the early 1910s, it was a profession on the defensive. Few people really understood its purpose. Supporters of the aspiring new profession did not need to explain the word "therapy;" most everyone agreed that the term meant some kind of treatment for either a mental or physical disorder. What had to be clarified was the use of the word "occupational." During the 1910s, most outsiders hearing the phrase "occupational therapy" interpreted it to denote "vocational." That is, they thought that occupational therapy patients (whom they called "invalids") would receive training in an appropriate field or vocation in order to be able to earn a living in spite of limitations due to illness. Although the founding generation agreed that work was an important prerequisite to good health, for "invalids" as well as anyone, their definition of occupational therapy was not simply vocational training. They held a holistic view of health, assuming that in order to achieve good health a patient had to engage body, mind, and spirit in the process of healing. Influenced by the arts and crafts and efficiency movements of the early 20th century, they argued that healing and good health came about when patients were systematically *occupied* with "meaningful" and "authentic" work, in particular, with craft activity. They instituted programs in which patients engaged in activities such as basketmaking, weaving, toymaking, or bookbinding. By interacting with individual patients the early occupational therapists learned that their treatments restored physical function, improved mental attitude, and in general, lessened suffering, thus quickening convalescence. Coming from a decidedly middle-class "therapeutic world view," as many progressive reformers did, these creators of occupational therapy argued that they directly addressed the health problems associated with modern life by combining the traditional values of the work ethic and crafts with scientific and medical principles.[4]

Yet, occupational therapy was on the defensive at its emergence in the early 20th century for at least two reasons: (1) occupational therapists believed that they had to fight the powerful world of scientific medicine in order to promote its holistic approaches to healthcare, and (2) occupational therapy was a new profession for *women*. Thus occupational therapy not only challenged early 20th-century mainstream medicine but also contemporary socially constructed gender roles. Most Americans still assumed that a woman's place was in the private domestic sphere or, if she entered healthcare, in nursing, as an assistant to a physician.

Many studies of women's work in charity organizations and professions have analyzed the cultural and ideological context in which middle- and upper-class women established a place for themselves outside the traditional sphere of marriage and family. Born in the last quarter of the 19th century, these women were members of what many historians have identified as a transitional generation of American women who transformed a late 19th-century legacy of women's charity and volunteer work into professional work in the early 20th century.[5] First charity workers and then aspiring professionals expanded the limits of 19th-century separate sphere ideology by arguing that women's moral superiority, natural nurturing qualities, and altruism could and should be applied beyond the private family for the good of society. In a world rapidly changing from a rural to an urban context and from an agricultural to an industrial base, socially conscious women fought to share in addressing the problems of modern society by improving conditions in the nation's schools, slums, hospitals, and social settlements. Fraught with conflict between traditional and modern female roles, many professional women of this transitional generation found that they could advance their influence on society by drawing on the strengths of women's networks as well as by aligning themselves with men in positions of authority. The women of Hull House in the 1890s, for example, expanded their financial base and political power and, by extension, their programs for social conscience by affiliating with female philanthropists and women's charity networks and male reformers and male-dominated institutions.[6] The founding generation of occupational therapists adopted this strategy as well. Slagle, who was part of the Hull House community in the early 20th century, spearheaded the effort.

Hull House, Mental Hygiene, Arts and Crafts, Education, and the Roots of Occupational Therapy

In the summer of 1911, Slagle began a lifelong labor of love, developing and promoting the new women's profession of occupational therapy. Slagle began her work by taking a course in "curative occupations and recreations" at the Chicago School of Civics and Philanthropy.[7] The course, an outgrowth of the mental hygiene movement, used state-of-the-art Progressive Era educational theory and methodology. It provided students with theoretical lectures, craft training, and practical clinical experience. The school itself was an offshoot of Chicago's Hull House Settlement, which served as a major recruiting and socializing agency, bringing aspiring young professional women into what historian Robyn Muncy calls "the female dominion in American reform."[8] Founded in 1889 by Jane Addams and Ellen Gates Starr, Hull House's secular community provided middle-class American women with a respectable alternative to marriage and family life, viable opportunities to become involved in public reform, and an important training ground for women's political and professional work. It also provided a fertile ground in which occupational therapy's beginnings would take root and thrive.

Hull House served as a meeting place for proponents of contemporary early 20th-century social movements that directly influenced the later development of occupational therapy. For example, in 1897 the Chicago Arts and Crafts Society organized at Hull House. There many middle- and upper-class Chicagoans and participated in this larger American and British movement by studying a variety of arts and crafts processes and thus resisting what they perceived to be the tyranny of the machine. At twice-monthly meetings the society aimed to revitalize and ennoble the meaning of work by recreating the ideal of the craftsperson in spite of the fact that society members lived in the machine age. Under the auspices of the society, for example, Starr held bookbinding classes in which "design and workmanship, beauty and thoroughness [were] taught to a small number of apprentices."[9]

Craftwork, as society members saw it, provided opportunities for them as nonworking-class people to capture what they perceived to be a productive and meaningful life experience. By actually using their hands, creating specimens of pottery, wood, glass, metal, or cloth, the members hoped to gain insight into the problem with which they struggled incessantly—alienation in modern life. In discussions, members analyzed and critiqued America's rapid and seemingly complete capitulation to "industrial organization and the machine," which had created a world in which they felt lost and aimless.[10]

In 1900, Addams and Starr, worried about workers' alienation and the problem of immigrant assimilation, created an educational institution called the Hull House Labor Museum, which subsequently spread the ideas and concerns of the arts and crafts movement to the working-class population of Chicago. The museum, financed by some wealthy Chicago women, primarily examined the history of textile production. Hoping to instill pride in immigrant women's textile-producing skills, Addams recruited Syrian, Greek, Italian, Russian, and Irish women to demonstrate spinning and weaving. Charts displayed on the wall illustrated the long history of hand labor in the making of threads, comparing the years of primacy of the stick spindle with the very brief period when the spinning wheel was used, and then with the era of steam-driven machines. At times, Addams displayed textile implements and tools, raw materials, and finished products.

To Addams, educational activities such as those offered by the Hull House Labor Museum helped alleviate tensions that workers experienced in modern industrial society. Influenced by the philosophy of contemporary Chicago educator John Dewey, an advocate of learning by doing or by actual experience, Addams believed that if workers learned the "history and growth of industrial processes," they would feel more connected to and less hostile toward factory processes of labor.[11] Addams brought workers to the museum to be "entertained, to work with the tools with which they are already familiar, to study charts and diagrams which are simple and graphic, to attend lectures which may illustrate their daily work, and give them some clew [sic] to the development of the machine and the materials which they constantly handle."[12]

Such a program, Addams claimed, conceived of education in terms that Dewey would call "a continuing reconstruction of experience."[13]

Occupational therapists grafted many ideas and practices from the arts and crafts and education reform movements as the new profession flourished. Practitioners vigorously adopted craft work and experiential learning as central practices in the field because they also valued authentic experience and productivity, as did other reformers. Like many of the leaders of the arts and crafts and education reform movements, occupational therapists came from middle- or upper-class segments of American society. Most, in addition, were educated, white, Protestant, and urban, as were their reformer counterparts. Because many of the tasks inherent in arts and crafts and education, such as weaving and teaching young children, were extensions of traditional women's work, women were well represented in these reform movements. Occupational therapy combined the skills of craftwork and teaching with those of caring for society's ill or needy—all of which were defined as proper women's work— thus occupational therapy would be a field highly dominated by women. Occupational therapists, that is, women with professional ambitions, would also draw financial support from wealthy women as did Addams.

By the 1910s, arts and crafts ideology, education reform, and women's assumed natural capacity to help so-called invalids merged, creating the basis of the new profession of occupational therapy. This, however, does not explain why the field was defined as a "therapy." Julia Lathrop, involved in the mental hygiene movement, created the connection between arts and crafts, education, and mental health care. Profoundly moved by the life experience of Clifford Beers, who wrote the book *A Mind That Found Itself*,[14] which launched mental hygiene into a nationwide movement, Lathrop was determined to reform the care and treatment of the mentally ill.

Collaborating with Graham Taylor, a Chicago leader of the settlement movement and head of the Chicago School of Civics and Philanthropy, Lathrop started experimental classes at the school. As Taylor phrased it, the course was "to train institution attendants in occupations for the insane." The course emphasized "the *educational* as opposed to the *custodial* idea in the daily care of the mentally unsound [emphasis in original].[15] A report that Taylor gave at the National Conference of Charities and Correction on the success of the first course helped attract hospital attendants from Indiana, New York, and other states during the next few years.[16] Slagle later praised the 6-week course for stimulating national interest in what she called "the normalizing effect of occupational work."[17]

Aspiring Professional Eleanor Clarke Slagle: The Preassociation Years

Slagle took the course in curative occupations when she was about 40 years old, but she had been imbued with the values of reform since childhood. Her character was shaped by an early life in rural upstate New York, where she discovered the importance of hard work and civic responsibility by observing her own immediate and extended family. Born circa 1871 in Hobart, New York, Ella May Clark, as she was then known, was the younger of two children and the only daughter of William John Clark, a cooper and later a sheriff of Delaware County, and Emmaline J. (Davenport) Clark.[18] The Clark and Davenport families had settled in Delaware County in the early 18th century and were well known. Emmaline was related to John Davenport, one of the founders of Yale University. Many Clarks and Davenports were active abolitionists, and several of the men in both families served in the Union Army during the Civil War. The marriage between William Clark and Emmaline Davenport took place shortly after William returned from serving as a second lieutenant in the New York Infantry during the Civil War. According to one source (left by their daughter-in-law Marian W. Clarke), William was 36 years old when he married; Emmaline was only 16. She gave birth first to a son, John Davenport Clark, in 1869 and then to Ella May 2 years later, bearing both before she reached the age of twenty.[19]

The members of Slagle's family in her early childhood followed traditional late 19th-century gender roles. Father William was reportedly a "strict disciplinarian with a rigid adherence to a firm sense of right and wrong"; mother Emmaline was a "soft and frivolous woman" who spoiled her son and daughter.[20] In certain ways, John and Ella May were treated equally: they were baptized together at St. Peter's Episcopal Church in Hobart on New Year's Eve in 1876, and they both attended private school at the Delaware Academy at nearby Delhi, New York. John had many more educational opportunities than his sister, however. He finished high school at Phillips Academy in Andover, Massachusetts, in 1894, and then went on to college in Colorado and to law school in Brooklyn, New York.[21] Ella May attended Hudson River Institute, Claverack College's high school program located near Hudson, New York, in 1885 and 1886, where she studied music, but she never attended college in a degree-granting program. The school nonetheless instilled in Ella May an urge to be civically responsible: it aimed to inculcate "refined manners, elevated social character, cultivated taste, and Christian morals" in its students.[22] A coeducational institution, Hudson River Institute may also have helped to prepare Ella May to work comfortably with men, which she later did with seeming ease and grace.

Slagle left no personal papers; thus many gaps in her personal history cannot be filled. Historians know little of the period between her school days and her appearance in Chicago, for example. What is certain is that she married Robert E. Slagle, the son of the Reverend Peter and Mrs. Cordelia (Beam) Slagle of Chicago, at St. Peter's Episcopal Church in Hobart on April 19, 1894, and that the couple planned to make their home in Chicago.[23] What is unknown is what Robert Slagle did for a living; where and how Ella May and Robert met, whether or not the marriage was a happy one; whether there were ever any children; why the couple lived in St. Louis for some years; and whether the couple divorced. In 1937, Slagle described herself as a "long time widow," but a grandniece later contradicted that statement, saying that Slagle was divorced.[24]

Slagle apparently never spoke of the 17 years between her wedding and her appearance at the Chicago School for Civics and Philanthropy in 1911, so it is difficult to say precisely why she pursued a professional life in occupational therapy. There is evidence that she was involved in some way in reform work. In the early 1920s she wrote a resume that was headed by the following statement: "Covering a period of years of interest in the unfair social attitude toward the dependency of mentally and physically handicapped, followed by lectures on Social Economics by Professor Henderson, Chicago University, Jane Adams [sic], Hull House, Julia Lathrop, now of the Children's Bureau, I took up: . . . [the special course in 1911 and continued on in occupational therapy.]"[25]

The health history of Slagle's family provides grounds for speculation on why she became interested in occupational therapy. She was surrounded by disability and chronic illness from childhood to adulthood. In several instances she found it her duty to be the family caregiver, and this experience oddly enough prepared her for a career in working with persons who were sickly or disabled. Her father was probably ill throughout her life: he returned from the Civil War partially disabled, having been wounded by a gunshot to the neck.[26] No evidence exists of the injury's effect on his ability to function, and whether Slagle had to tend to him as a child or as a young woman is not known. She definitely assumed a caregiving role when he became ill in his later life, however. William Clark spent his final years with his married daughter in St. Louis, leaving his wife and his upstate New York home behind. The marriage apparently dissolved, Emmaline returning to her father's home with John.[27] Slagle's brother and her nephew, two other significant men in her life, suffered various ailments as well.

Seeing her father, brother, and nephew struggle with disabling injuries and debilitating illnesses may have been the personal experience that drove Slagle to the Chicago School of Civics and Philanthropy in 1911. Practically speaking, Slagle, as a single woman, needed to find a means to earn a living. Immediately upon completion of the course, which included both an academic focus and a field experience in which she studied Illinois hospitals and charitable institutions, Slagle procured employment in state hospitals in Michigan and New York, where she studied and organized "reeducation classes."[28]

Slagle worked with leaders of the mental hygiene movement. Already gaining a name for herself in the fledgling field of occupational therapy and having made connections with Chicago leaders of the mental hygiene movement, in 1912 Slagle went to Baltimore to direct a new department of occupational therapy in the Henry Phipps Psychiatric Clinic of Johns Hopkins Hospital, which was headed by psychiatrist Adolph Meyer, formerly of Illinois. In late 1913, Slagle attended the Maryland State Conference on Mental Hygiene, at which she met with her former colleague Taylor of the Chicago School of Civics and Philanthropy. Taylor visited the Phipps Clinic, which he described in a letter to Lathrop as "a wonderful place" that "impressively combined . . . work, science, and sympathy." Slagle, he told Lathrop, "besought" him to "renew . . . efforts to train others for the work she is so masterfully accomplishing and for which she thinks an increasing demand is sure to develop." Taylor not only saw the importance of occupational therapy in mental healthcare but found that it could be well applied in tuberculosis prevention and care. Taylor pressed Lathrop to continue working with him to educate occupational therapy workers in more than just mental hygiene.[29]

Slagle's lobbying of Taylor apparently paid off: by early 1914 she resigned her position at the Phipps Clinic to return to Chicago, the hotbed of reform. Back at the Chicago School of Civics and Philanthropy she gave lectures on occupations. More significantly, under the auspices of the Illinois Society for Mental Hygiene she started a workshop for the chronically unemployed, called the experimental station. Although the program was organized primarily for patients with mental illness, "the demand was so great," Slagle later wrote, "that all types . . . of borderline mental cases and orthopedic cripples . . . were admitted."[30] Soon she headed a school of occupational therapy named after a recently deceased Chicago physician, Henry B. Favill, who was one of the founders of the Chicago Anti-Tuberculosis Society and a leader in national mental hygiene as well.[31]

Slagle stayed in Chicago for the next few years, but she made it her business to contact people in other cities who began to see, as she did, that her work had the potential to become its own professional field. She nurtured the relationships that she forged with women and men involved in the mental hygiene and antituberculosis movements and with female philanthropists who would finance her projects, and she made new allies among hospital physicians, psychiatrists, and nurses who worked directly with patients. In particular, Slagle nurtured relationships with other practitioners of occupational therapy, such as nurse Susan Tracy, with whom she held many things in common. Both Slagle and Tracy first became acquainted with occupational therapy while working in psychiatry, which in itself was in a reform period. Other experiences bonded them as well, such as wanting to promote the use of occupational therapy, struggling to create a professional niche for themselves, and heading their own experiment stations in which they practiced occupational therapy. However, their ideas about where occupational therapy fit in the world of medicine diverged dramatically, as did the professional style and manner with which these women conducted themselves.

Susan E. Tracy and Nurses for Invalid Occupations

In 1910, when the American Society of Superintendents of Training Schools for Nurses met in New York City, nursing leader Adelaide Nutting of Teacher College, Columbia University, arranged for a special exhibition. This "Educational Museum," as she labeled it (note the similarity to Hull House's Labor Museum), displayed experimental work in the new field of "occupations for invalids." One of the participants, Boston-based physician Hall, showed handicrafts made by patients treated for "nervous exhaustion" at his small mental asylum in Marblehead, Massachusetts. The Chicago School of Civics and Philanthropy exhibited work by patients from Illinois mental hospitals. Tracy's exhibit, "The Testing of Invalid Occupations in the Adams Nervine Asylum, Jamaica Plain, Massachusetts," showed handcrafts made by patients and ways to instruct nurses in this new field.[32]

Susan E. Tracy was an important figure in the movement to promote occupational therapy in the first decades of the 20th century. Born in Lynn, Massachusetts, in 1878 and graduated from the Massachusetts Homeopathic Hospital Nursing school in 1898, she, like Slagle, was a member of the first generation of professional women in the United States.[33] Little is known of Tracy's family and personal life, partly because no unpublished personal or professional papers survived—thus it is difficult to analyze Tracy's motivations and ambitions in relation to nursing and occupational therapy. A few sources such as annual reports of hospitals, some patient case records, contemporary articles about Tracy's work, and a few of Tracy's own professional publications, however, provide a framework in which to examine her career. In 1906 she organized occupational therapy classes in her training school for nurses at the Adams Nervine Asylum. She trained practitioners not only in the Boston area but in Chicago and New York. In 1910 she published a textbook that was widely used in the field until at least 1940.[34] Another important contribution that Tracy made to the field was to take occupational therapy from its limited place in psychiatric institutions to the homes of patients, an important locus of care in the early 20th century. Her contemporaries in nursing and occupational therapy considered her a pioneer in advancing women's professional work.[35]

Many of Tracy's colleagues who were interested in developing occupational therapy as an independent profession, however, had ambivalent feelings about the nursing pioneer. Tracy wanted to establish occupational therapy as a subspecialty of nursing; other leaders of the occupational therapy movement disagreed. Slagle and Susan Cox Johnson, both founders of the National Society for the Promotion of Occupational Therapy, acknowledged that practitioners needed coursework in medicine, as nurses did. Johnson, coming from the perspective of a teacher, argued that "occupations teachers," as she called them, needed grounding in pedagogy and sociology too.[36] Eventually the will and viewpoints of the other founders became the norm: occupational therapy found its own identity separate from nursing but including the perspectives of several other fields. Yet, to examine the career of Tracy illustrates the short-lived link between occupational therapy and nursing, the struggle within occupational therapy to define its professional boundaries, and the ambivalence of early 20th century American women in declaring themselves as professionals.

Tracy at the Adams Nervine Asylum

Susan E. Tracy formally began her work in "invalid occupations" at the Adams Nervine Asylum in Jamaica Plain, Massachusetts, a small mental institution founded in the late 19th century. The Adams Nervine Asylum catered to "nervous invalids" rather than to persons who were seriously mentally ill, according to the resident physician Daniel H. Fuller.[37] Specifically, most of the patients at the Adams Nervine Asylum suffered from "neurasthenia," a newly identified illness. Late 19th-century physicians declared that the illness was caused by the stresses of modern life. People had limited energy; when they were taxed by overwork, stress, or strain in the marketplace or at home, one or more of the bodily systems broke down, provoking neurasthenia. Complete bed rest and a bland diet, to the point of infantilization, offered the only hope of restoring the exhausted patient to health. This so-called rest cure was popularized by elite Philadelphia physician S. Weir Mitchell.[38] At the Adams Nervine Asylum around the turn of the century the rest cure dominated the therapy program.

Caught up in broad reforms that called for psychiatry to become more aggressive in its therapies, many psychiatrists after 1900 began to criticize the rest cure. Meyer's ideas had influenced many American psychiatrists to view patients as mentally ill if they were unable to function well in their environment. Such patients, the theory went, had been debilitated by certain defective habits learned early in life that prevented them from adapting to adulthood. Meyer believed that patients with mental illness could be cured by "habit training" regimens that would restore them to a balanced, healthful life.[39]

By the first decade of the 20th century the staff at the Adams Nervine Asylum had also renounced the rest cure, exchanging its near custodialism for more active therapies. A chapter authored by Fuller in Tracy's book, *Studies in Invalid Occupation,* described a multitude of approaches used at the Adams Nervine Asylum, among them drugs; massage; electricity; gymnastics; dietary regimens; hydrotherapy; light, heat, and fresh air; occupations; instruction in methods of self-help; and suggestion or psychotherapy.[40]

Fuller saw many advantages in engaging his "nervous invalid" patients in occupations. Like Meyer, he believed that occupations diverted attention from illness and established new and healthier life habits. The occupations room created a "new environment," taking patients away from their "individual apartment" filled with the "suggestion of invalidism." Occupations also offered a "means of switching the attention from morbid introspection to . . . normal interests, . . . excluding abnormal habits of mind."[41]

Fuller hired Tracy in 1905, and for the next 7 years she supervised the nursing school, developed the occupations program with Fuller, and conducted several postgraduate courses for nurses. Later, Fuller wrote that he had "secured an excellent leader, [who was both] trained in teaching and conversant with the work to be taken up."[42] Fuller clearly realized that nurses trained in occupations were necessary in helping him to carry out his crusade against the rest cure.

Although Fuller may have thought that both he and his nurse were involved in the intellectual exercise of reforming psychiatry, Tracy held a different attitude toward the work she was doing. In contrast to Fuller's reliance on theoretical reasons why occupations ought to be practiced, Tracy claimed that she based her approach on mere common sense and observation. She had spent 7 years in private duty nursing before going to the Adams Nervine Asylum. That experience had convinced her that patients were "happier when their hands and minds were occupied."[43] Even though she had studied at Teachers College, taking courses in crafts and hospital economics, she never acknowledged any formal training beyond traditional nursing school. She modestly said that she had learned many crafts in childhood and that when she became a nurse and "found herself responsible for removing the tedium of lagging hours," she reverted to occupations learned at her mother's side.[44]

Unlike psychiatrists, Tracy never attempted theoretical explanations about when one ought to practice occupational therapy, nor did she feel the need to understand why one should. She simply designed a practical curriculum for her students at the Adams Nervine Asylum that would prepare them to work with patients with neurasthenia as well as with the variety of cases that they would face when they graduated to become private duty nurses. Her textbook was dominated by practical discussions of craft projects for convalescents of various age, sex, class, and medical categories. Each of her lessons required students to make a craft article, blending their arts and crafts skills with the medical knowledge that they had acquired in other courses. Her greatest concern was to develop judgment skills in students so that they could select appropriate activities for the patients.[45]

Speaking from her own experience, Tracy declared that only nurses should practice occupations, for only they understood the limitations that different diseases impose and the positive and negative consequences that various activities could produce. Nurses were able to notice "eye strain" and "fatigue" even before the patient became aware of them. Nurses were also able to recognize nervous disorders and temperamental differences among patients, and only nurses could produce individualized work plans to address these conditions, she claimed.[46] Tracy tried to make patient occupations a specialty within nursing, even offering a few courses at Teachers College in the early 1910s.[47] If nothing more, she hoped that the training in occupations would provide practitioners with skills that would ease the burdens of their daily practice. In offering the training, Tracy spoke to a problem that nursing leaders recognized: private duty nursing was physically and psychologically exhausting.[48]

When speaking of Tracy in public, colleagues in psychiatry and nursing described her as a "caring" nurse devoted to serving society. They carefully commended her for contributing to nursing and occupational therapy while never projecting an image that in the least way might make her look self-interested, commercial, or "unladylike." Maryland psychiatrist Dunton, a strong supporter of occupational therapy and the editor of the *Maryland Psychiatric Quarterly*, devoted an entire issue to her work in occupations. In that issue he praised her for organizing the "first systematic training course for nurses in occupations" at the Adams Nervine Asylum, yet he deliberately wrote with restraint because he did not want to "embarrass the dear lady."[49] Another contributor to the special issue described interviewing Tracy in her home, depicted it as an environment of domestic grace. Tracy reportedly greeted the writer at the door with "outstretched hands" and then "conducted [the writer] into her quaint old-fashioned home" with a "huge fireplace in the sitting room," for a meeting in which Tracy stated that she had decided to "devote the rest of her life to occupational therapy."[50]

Such mythologizing of Tracy can best be understood in the context of the history of nursing and the general predicament in which professional women found themselves in the early 20th century. Tracy entered nursing during a period of reform in which leaders were struggling to gain recognition and power for the profession. Susan Reverby has argued that professionalization presented several dilemmas to superintendent leaders in nursing. Nurses were caught in a trap in which they were expected to maintain a particularly feminine form of a service ethic, and furthermore, they were usually idealized as women with "natural" characters of self-sacrifice and patience. Moreover, nurses were caught between traditional views of the "caring" nurse and the needs of hospital authorities moving toward efficient and scientific approaches to the care of patients. Nurses needed to "know" more; thus the profession pressed for higher educational criteria. Yet, this greater knowledge did not guarantee nursing an authoritative position in the evolving medical hierarchy of the early 20th century.[51] Tracy could not escape many of these quandaries.

Women aspiring to careers in Tracy's generation had to make it clear that their motives were based on altruism and service to society. If they held personal ambitions for or intellectual interests in work outside their traditional family duties, they rarely made public declarations of these motives. Such declarations would not have been socially acceptable. Rather, they commonly mythologized their calling to professional work by telling stirring stories of it: for example, Addams's tale of being inspired to found the Hull House Settlement in 1889 after seeing the "wretchedness of east London" and the innovative work at Toynbee Hall[52] and Lillian Wald's account of starting the Henry Street Settlement in New York City after witnessing the misery in the lower east side's immigrant neighborhoods.[53]

Women of the founding generation of occupational therapy told such stories as well. Slagle claimed to have received her "inspiration and incentive" to work in occupational therapy during a "chance visit" to the Kankakee State Hospital in Illinois while she was studying at the Chicago School of Civics and Philanthropy. In fact, she was conducting a study of the institution to determine the state of patients' care, as were other mental hygiene reformers such as Lathrop. Slagle told how she noticed an "unkempt young" female patient unraveling her knitted underclothing from her waist in order to make a little shirt for a child. Slagle spoke to the women, asking if she was making the garment for her daughter. The patient's "face lighted," so the story goes, and she exclaimed "that she actually had four children." Slagle left that day determined to help overcome the "appalling idleness of the mentally sick in the institutions [which was] a constant degenerating influence." When she repeated this story years later, she made sure to include the fact that some "Chicago women" helped her to establish a community workshop under the auspices of the Illinois Society for Mental Hygiene, where persons with physical and mental disabilities were trained in occupations.[54]

Tracy, too, mythologized her calling to occupations. She described her days as a student nurse at the Massachusetts Homeopathic Hospital, where she had noticed that surgical patients who kept busy working managed to maintain their spirits. One courageous woman spent every last minute until surgery embroidering. Another woman recovered rapidly from abdominal surgery while lying on her back crocheting an elaborate piece of trimming. A young girl kept herself and others in the ward lively while she worked on projects in spite of the fact that one of her legs had been amputated.[55] Tracy told and retold these anecdotes, thus explaining why she had become interested in occupations. More important, she accounted for her leadership in the field: it was all for the benefit of patients.

The Experiment Station for the Study of Invalid Occupations

The image of Tracy as a self-sacrificing lady and nurse suggests that she lived up to the cultural roles expected of turn-of-the-century American women. Yet,

Tracy was more than the demure lady that she chose to portray. In 1912 she broke her ties with the Adams Nervine Asylum to set up her own institution, which she called the Experiment Station for the Study of Invalid Occupations. In the Jamaica Plain, Massachusetts, location she instructed patients and public health and graduate nurses. She also created a resource center, claiming to keep complete records of all work done in the field.

One observer interpreted Tracy's leaving of the Adams Nervine Asylum as its having been thrust on her because of lack of space.[56] In actuality, Tracy planned the move years before. In a 1910 speech to the American Society of Superintendents of Training Schools for Nurses she called for setting up "a bureau" for training "occupations nurses" in every large city so that nurses could gain control over practice. From their respective experiment stations, she argued, skilled occupations nurses could be sent patients "of all sorts and conditions" to practice their specialization.[57]

In establishing the Experiment Station, Tracy sought to establish autonomy and independence for herself and other nurses who desired self-sufficiency in their workplaces and freedom from the confines of physician-dominated hospitals. Her true motive was to upgrade nurses' status by providing them with specialized skills. Although she may have claimed to be disinterested in theory, her establishment of the resource center, where she collected case studies for others to examine, proves her interest in gathering a body of knowledge. For Tracy, however, that knowledge was to be based in experience or practice, not theory. Did she leave the Adams Nervine Asylum in frustration because her way of thinking about patient care went unappreciated? More likely, she simply needed to free herself from the responsibilities of her nursing superintendency in order to create more opportunities for spreading the occupational therapy gospel.

Tracy influenced many nurses in the first 2 decades of the 20th century, converting many of them to the cause, and in doing so she, in effect, transported the practice of occupational therapy from its original, limited place in psychiatric institutions to many other arenas in which medicine was practiced. The nurses whom she trained at the Adams Nervine Asylum later practiced in the homes of patients, using occupational therapy to treat patients with physical as well as mental illness. Many of her students went on to establish their own institutions of practice or to head occupational therapy departments in hospitals as such departments slowly increased in number during the 1910s. Her visits to many other institutions, to give single lectures or complete courses to student and postgraduate nurses, ensured such a process. In 1911, for example, she gave lessons to the senior class at the nursing school at Massachusetts General Hospital. By 1916 she had given courses at the

Newton and Children's Hospitals in Boston and the Michael Reese and Rush-Presbyterian hospitals in Chicago, and she had lectured several times at Teachers College in New York, among other places. That year she taught a 3-month course at Teachers College, dividing classes between ward patients and student nurses.[58]

Tracy did not attend the founding meeting of the National Society for the Promotion of Occupational Therapy, opting instead to commit her time to training newcomers to the field. While the founders met in upstate New York, she instead taught "occupations courses" for nurses in Chicago at the Rush Presbyterian and Michael Reese Hospitals. In spite of her absence her peers acknowledged her pioneering work in the field, declaring her an honorary founding member. In recognition of the 1906 course she ran at the Adams Nervine Asylum they elected her to the position of chair of the Committee on Teaching Methods.[59] During the next 5 years, Tracy contributed several papers on teaching to the national association.[60]

Yet, Tracy's absence from the founder's meeting in 1917 accurately pointed to the widening gap between herself and other leaders in occupational therapy. Tracy never saw occupational therapy become a subspecialty within nursing. Until her death in 1928, Tracy saw few occupational therapy departments or teaching institutions headed by nurses, although in many cases, nurses worked alongside occupational therapists, many of whom received their training during World War I. Leaders and promoters of occupational therapy opened many emergency schools during the war in major American cities such as Boston, Chicago, Milwaukee, New York, Philadelphia, and St. Louis, drawing applicants who identified themselves as nurses, teachers, artists, craftswomen, and attendants. A severe wartime shortage of nurses also accelerated the growth of nursing schools, but few, if any, included training in occupations. Such training was confined to schools for "reconstruction aides," the wartime name for occupational and physical therapists who were involved in the movement to "reconstruct" wounded soldiers and sailors returning from the front.[61]

However, Tracy's ideas of establishing independent institutions for practice, and recruiting new students, and mentoring them into leadership roles in the developing profession caught hold among her colleagues in cities all over the nation. Indeed, leaders of many of the war emergency schools focused their time and attention on keeping their newly established schools open and growing. Those institutions that survived after the war served as centers of occupational therapy's professional development and culture, just as the Hull House Settlement had fueled the growth of many women's professions in

Chicago decades before. The obvious leader to take the new profession through this phase was Slagle, the woman most capable of dwelling in two worlds: medicine and the culture of women's reform.

The Consummate Professional:
Eleanor Clarke Slagle in the Association Years

Central to occupational therapy's growth and success during the late 1910s and early 1920s was the role played by the National Society for the Promotion of Occupational Therapy. During World War I, the organization had served as a clearinghouse of information on domestic and overseas reconstruction efforts, domestic training programs, and shifts in federal government policy. Following the war, the association concentrated efforts on stabilizing growth and development and standardizing education and practice standards. Members of the organization exchanged information, shared ideas, developed strategies to promote the field, and debated issues critical to occupational therapy's further development. Conference attendance soared: whereas fewer than 10 persons participated in the founding meeting, in Clifton Springs, New York, in March 1917, nearly 300 attended the third annual meeting in Chicago in the fall of 1919.[62]

By the time the membership met in Chicago in 1919 many idealistically felt that the profession had achieved acceptance by the general public and medicine. Dunton declared that occupational therapy was "coming into its own."[63] At the next annual meeting, President Eleanor Clarke Slagle optimistically discussed removing the word "promotion" from the name of the group.[64] In 1921, with new self-assurance the membership voted to change the organization's name from the National Society for the Promotion of Occupational Therapy to the American Occupational Therapy Association. During 1920 the journal *Modern Hospital* launched a regular column on occupational therapy. In 1921 the association started its own professional journal, the *Archives of Occupational Therapy,* under the editorship of Dunton.[65]

On the other hand, the overwhelmingly female membership was not completely convinced that occupational therapy had acquired legitimacy. During these early years a pattern of electing men to the office of the president emerged. Further, with the exceptions of George Edward Barton (1917) and Thomas B. Kidner (1923–28), both of whom held close connections to World War rehabilitation circles, all the men elected were physicians. Only one woman served as president before World War II—Eleanor Clarke Slagle (1919–1920), after a very close election.

Johnson, chair of the 1919 elections committee, articulated the problem in simple language. She told the membership that the committee recommended Hall for the office of the president because he was "one of the leading physicians interested in occupational therapy" and active in the field. Furthermore, she said, "placing a physician as president will have the tendency to stimulate interest and confidence on the part of physicians in general, and emphasize the therapeutic purpose of our work." The committee slated Slagle for the vice presidency, but members of the association nominated her for the presidency as well. When the votes were counted, Slagle had fifteen to Hall's thirteen.[66]

Slagle certainly possessed the organizational skills and the self-confidence to preside over the neophyte association. For nearly a decade before her nomination for the presidency she had worked indefatigably in the field. After completing her course at the Chicago School of Civics and Philanthropy in 1911 she conducted a 6-month survey of the care of patients with mental illness and then organized a school of occupational therapy for nurses, attendants, and patients at the Upper Peninsula State Hospital in Newberry, Michigan. From there she accepted employment at the state hospital in Central Islip, Long Island, to organize reeducation classes under the auspices of the Russell Sage Foundation. In 1914 she went to the Phipps Clinic, staying for 2 years before returning to Chicago. In 1916 she took a summer leave to attend courses at Columbia University's Teachers College in New York City. By 1917 she had taken the position of general superintendent of occupational therapy for all the state hospitals in Illinois. Then, after turning down at least two offers to serve in reconstruction work in Washington she directed a war emergency school at the Chicago School of Civics and Philanthropy, called the Henry B. Favill School of Occupations.[67]

Without a doubt, Slagle had adopted a professional persona modeled after her Hull House colleagues Addams and Lathrop. She saw many Chicago women take positions of authority in their fields, so it is no surprise that she internalized self-assurance in pursuing professional work. Perhaps not coincidentally, Slagle was elected to the presidency of the National Society during the third annual meeting, held at Hull House in Chicago. On the very day that Slagle won the election, Addams addressed the membership on the topic of mental hygiene and its relationship to occupational therapy.[68] Women's rightful authority in professional work permeated the national meeting in 1919.

That authority was fleeting, however, at least as far as its being expressed through the presidency of the organization. At the next annual meeting, in 1920, psychiatrist Hall won the office after another close race with Slagle. Although Slagle felt strongly enough about taking authority in her chosen vocation to compete for the highest leadership position in 1919 and 1920, she never ran for the presidency again.

For the next 15 years, Slagle served as secretary-treasurer, a position she made sure wielded great power. In her role as secretary-treasurer she traveled extensively all over the country to speak and to launch dozens of new occupational therapy schools and occupational therapy departments in hospitals and private institutions. Occupational therapy lore has it that although Slagle was no longer the official head of the association, she was nonetheless its heart and soul. In 1922 she moved to New York, the state in which she was born and in which her family still resided. In New York City she established the headquarters of the American Occupational Therapy Association, where it remained for years because Slagle was there to run the majority of its business.[69]

Slagle had exercised skills in grassroots recruiting, mentioning, and networking in order to promote occupational therapy while she lived and worked in Baltimore and in the Midwest. When she returned to New York, she perfected the skills into a system. She interacted with individual colleagues, she mentored new recruits, and most important, she networked with club women to promote the field. Slagle understood the crucial role that women's clubs had played in the promotion of women's professional work in Chicago and in other places, and she planned to continue cooperative relationships with organized womanhood to help occupational therapy in the years to come.

She invited collaboration from women club leaders whom she knew through her family's earlier philanthropic activities. President Hewitt of the New York State Federation of Women's Clubs, according to Slagle, had known her even before she identified herself as a professional woman. Hewitt worked with Slagle because she believed that the National Society for the Promotion of Occupational Therapy and the New York State Federation of Women's Clubs shared aims. Hewitt and her 275,000 members were committed to tackling problems in child welfare, public health, education, and what she called "humanity," or promoting "better ways and means for the betterment of . . . defectives, misfits, and unfortunates." At the annual meeting of the National Society for the Promotion of Occupational Therapy in 1920, Hewitt told members that the General Federation of Women's Clubs, with its two million newly enfranchised women, would bring "spiritual" and political power to the movement. She pledged the club women's vote to help pass federal bills to provide funding for the "humanitarian" and "good business" aims of bringing "human souls" back "to the plane of independent action."[70]

Slagle followed up immediately on the offer of collaboration with the General Federation of Women's Clubs. In late fall 1920 she took the position of chair of the Committee on Occupational Therapy, Division of Health, General Federation of Women's Clubs. Her duties involved educating women to use occupational therapy in hospital and community activities across the nation. Between this position and her position in the American Occupational Therapy Association, Slagle was able to use her influence to organize new clinics and workshops all over the United States.

In 1921, Slagle interacted with several Junior League and General Federation of Women's Clubs state chapters, using grassroots organizing methods. She advised Junior League groups setting up workshops in Detroit, Michigan; Bridgeport and Stamford, Connecticut; and the Oranges, New Jersey. She gathered lecture fees for club talks and donated them to build a state organization of occupational therapists in New York. At Ogdensburg, New York, she urged Northern New York Federation of Women's Club members to raise funds to send students to training schools.[71]

Slagle was as comfortable in speaking at various medical profession meetings as she was in working with the women's clubs. In 1921 she organized a group of speakers and an exhibition for the annual meeting of the National Tuberculosis Association. Male associates Dr. Philip King Brown and Hall supported the cause by giving talks on occupational therapy at the meeting. Hall and Slagle both appeared at the annual meeting of the American Psychiatric Association, he speaking on financial considerations and she on starting new departments of occupational therapy from the viewpoint of the practitioner. That year Slagle wrote plans for two large tuberculosis sanatoriums in Tennessee and Indiana. She also toured the country to give keynote talks at the launchings of at least six state associations and training schools.[72] During 1922, Slagle continued her networking by visiting several state occupational therapy associations, other medical associations, schools, women's clubs, and hospitals in Wisconsin, Illinois, Indiana, Ohio, the District of Columbia, and Minnesota, where, according to a later comment, she met William Mayo of the famous Mayo Clinic.[73]

All this while she held down the office of secretary-treasurer. In 1922 she relocated the office to a building where other health professions conducted business. (Previously, Slagle had handled most association business from her own apartment, keeping all official files in a packing box in the kitchen.) That year she regularly corresponded with medical authorities all over the country;

she singlehandedly conducted a placement service for practitioners, naming sixty-seven candidates for positions; and she received dues and sent routine correspondence to the association members. She also sent 3,805 invitations to the planned Sixth Annual Meeting of the American Occupational Therapy Association in Atlantic City, New Jersey, where the American Hospital Association was scheduled to meet concurrently.[74]

Conclusions

This examination of the careers of Susan E. Tracy and Eleanor Clarke Slagle and their contributions to the history and development of occupational therapy has provided a lens through which we can understand varied experiences of the pioneer generation of women professionals in the United States. In the context of American ambivalence toward women who stepped out of traditional roles into professional work, we have seen how Tracy and Slagle balanced differently the images of altruistic lady and independent professional as they traversed the cultural transformation which more and more accepted public roles for women. Both women claimed that their calling to nursing and occupational therapy was based upon altruism, yet they simultaneously sought autonomy and independence for themselves and their respective fields.

Although we may never know exactly what led Tracy to nursing, limited evidence suggests that she identified with the widespread service ethic that attracted so many women of her generation to professional work. Perhaps Tracy consciously chose not to marry in order to dedicate herself to such work unimpeded, but this is another question we will not be able to answer definitively; nor will we know the names and vocations of her mentors or what particular childhood influences sparked her attraction to nursing as her chosen field.

What is very clear, however, is that unlike Slagle, Tracy balked at certain norms of professional behavior. She did not feel comfortable in making public arguments on behalf of the profession of occupational therapy. For example, as the debate raged over whether the rest cure ought to be replaced by occupational therapy, Tracy deliberately stayed out of the fray. In spite of her years of work with psychiatric patients, her public writings leave no record of participation in such controversial theoretical discussions. For Tracy, embracing Meyer's psychobiological approach to psychiatric care, as did her colleague Slagle, was not essential to creating effective practice. She, instead, emphasized the development of experience-based practice.

Slagle, on the other hand, with the influence she exercised, eventually persuaded a whole generation of occupational therapists to employ Meyer's habit-training regimen. Slagle wanted physicians to see that her field identified with scientific medicine because unlike nursing, occupational therapy had to create a demand for itself. By the early 20th century few physicians doubted the vital role nurses played in the care of patients, whereas occupational therapists still had to convince most physicians of the value of their work. If occupational therapy did not take on a medical identity, it would remain in the marginal world of the projects of the women's auxiliaries in hospitals. Thus Slagle steered the profession toward medicine, insisting by the early 1920s that practitioners demand prescriptions from physicians for the patients they sent to the occupational therapy departments. Practitioners and patients, she said, "must have the protection of the prescription [emphasis in original]." With prescriptions from physicians, occupational therapists could take on the role of modern health care professionals. Procuring such a legitimate place in medicine distanced them from the do-gooder image of the earlier practitioners who came to the hospital under the auspices of volunteer charity programs.[75] Slagle realized that allying her profession with the needs of physicians was a necessity for the survival of occupational therapy, and she had no trouble acting upon such a plan.

Tracy also differed with Slagle over the primacy of the national association. While Slagle concentrated on the business of the national association, Tracy focused her energy and loyalty on strengthening local institutions such as her experiment station. In part, Tracy eluded continued involvement with the association because as time passed she realized that she was a nurse first and not an occupational therapist. However, her disregard for the association was not unique. After World War I, and well into the 1920s the occupational therapy workforce was heterogeneous, made up of arts and crafts instructors (mainly working in mental hospitals), emergency-trained reconstruction aides, and a handful of college-educated practitioners. Many of these practitioners did not identify themselves as occupational therapy professionals, thus they saw no reason to involve themselves with the association. For example, many of the reconstruction aides left the field as soon as the war emergency was over.[76] For others, who had experienced the heady days of helping reconstruct soldiers, sailors, and other patients with chronic illness, the top priority became strengthening existing local institutions for training and practice. Loyalty to peers, mentors, school, and workplace undergirded their activities. Volunteerism, social connections, female camaraderie, fundraising, public relations efforts, and sheer will kept many an institution afloat during this pivotal period in occupational therapy's history. Slowly, however, leaders realized that they had to transcend such a local focus to ensure the profession's growth and development; isolated practitioners had to be persuaded to identify with the aims of the profession at large. Eventually, members of the occupational therapy movement organized on the state or regional level. Some even concerned themselves with national issues, overcoming a widespread indifference toward the American Occupational Therapy Association.

In the critical decade of the 1920s, Slagle spent most of her energy building the profession from the inside as well as working with the men involved in the movement who concentrated on convincing outsiders of the value of occupational therapy. Hall, Kidner, and C. Floyd Haviland held the presidency of the American Occupational Therapy Association during the 1920s. These men moved in prominent circles of psychiatry, rehabilitation, and care of persons with tuberculosis, respectively, and were key to making sure that occupational therapy played important roles in these medical specialties.

During the 1920s, occupational therapy stabilized its professional identity. To accomplish this goal, occupational therapy gained control over practice and practitioners by standardizing practice and curriculum, establishing entry and exit criteria for schools, and expanding opportunities in the care of persons with chronic illness. Further, the profession created and nurtured a well-trained elite corps of leaders. Also crucial in this period was the strengthening of communication between the American Occupational Therapy Association and other organized medical groups: the American Hospital Association, the American Medical Association, the National Tuberculosis Association, and more. Using such linkages, the first generation of occupational therapists, allied with their male supporters, set the profession squarely in a medical model.[77]

However, occupational therapists—as exemplified by the career of Slagle—continued to dwell in the two worlds of medicine and the culture of women's reform. They straddled these worlds in part because the work that they were doing did not fit comfortably into the world of scientific medicine. Perhaps this is why Tracy was reluctant to pursue what other contemporary healthcare professions found imperative, creating a precise body of knowledge based upon scientific theory. Practice, to her, involved attracting patients' attention to craftwork, teaching patients the skills necessary to conduct such work, and supervising patients' progress through such activities. She knew that craftwork made it difficult for practitioners to demonstrate tangible improvement in patients, at least by the standards of scientific medicine. Rather than struggle to find methods of producing "objective" evidence, then, many first-generation occupational therapists persisted in embracing the experiential and practical traditions begun in the Hull House Labor Museum decades before. Slagle's organizational talents in convincing both medical colleagues and women's reform constituents that occupational therapy was a valid and efficacious treatment and an appropriate professional field for women helped to insure its continued growth. Of all the leaders of the first generation of occupational therapy, Slagle embodied the combination of women's reform and scientific values and ideas that set occupational therapy on its professional trajectory. An influential woman, Slagle largely shaped the profession of occupational therapy, helping to keep in balance its many disciplinary aspects internally while skillfully fixing connections to outside supporters.

As Slagle retired in 1937, she passed the torch on to the next generation of practitioners. The second generation of occupational therapists had certain values and orientations in common with its predecessors. They used crafts in therapy, and they maintained relationships with women's clubs and reform organizations. Although they had to learn to negotiate with a medical world that held increasing power over hospital policy, many independent institutions of practice and training continued to thrive because of the support of women's networks.

Unlike the first generation, practitioners trained in the 1920s and later never needed to ask themselves if they were teachers, nurses, or craftswomen, and certainly, they knew they were not in the category of volunteer altruist. Their professional identity was intact. Personal ambivalence over the role of women in professional work may have changed as well. After World War II, female practitioners took over the position of president in the American Occupational Therapy Association previously held by male physicians, blurring the gender-defined division of labor instituted by the first generation. Occupational therapy had truly become "a new profession for women."

VIRGINIA METAXAS, PhD
Professor of History and Women's Studies
Southern Connecticut State University
501 Cresscent Street
New Haven, Connecticut 06515

Acknowledgments

Portions of this article are excerpted from the introduction and chapters 1, 3, and 8 of Virginia A. Metaxas Quiroga's Occupational Therapy: The First Thirty

Years 1900–1930 *(Baltimore, Md.: American Occupational Therapy Association, 1995). Copyright 1995 by the American Occupational Therapy Association, Inc. Reprinted by permission of the American Occupational Therapy Association. A brief version of this paper, "Nurses for invalid occupations," was presented at the national meeting of the American Association of the History of Medicine, Seattle, Wash., 1992. I want to thank members of my New York City history writer's group including Polly Beals, Lucy Bowditch, Jane Covell, and Cynthia Ward, and my colleague Janet L. Golden for suggestions on earlier drafts.*

Notes

1. By 1922 the National Society for the Promotion of Occupational Therapy was renamed the American Occupational Therapy Association.

2. My concept of the early 20th-century American culture of professionalism is based on the work of Burton J. Bledstein, *The Culture of Professionalism: The Middle Class and the Development of Higher Education in America* (New York: W.W. Norton and Company, 1976). I have also used Bledstein's definition of the term profession, which he describes as a vocation requiring specialized knowledge in some area of learning or science. Furthermore, according to Bledstein, to achieve status in the professional community, members must be trained in the science and the techniques needed for practice. Professional knowledge is exclusive in order to eliminate the possibility of outsiders infringing on professional rights. Typically, training and membership in professional organizations instill a professional conscience and a group solidarity. For a description of American medicine's gradual evolution toward science and technology, see Paul Starr, *The Social Transformation of American Medicine: The Rise of a Sovereign Profession and the Making of a Vast Industry* (New York: Basic Books, 1982).

3. Virginia A. Metaxas Quiroga, *Occupational Therapy: The First Thirty Years 1900–1930* (Baltimore, Md.: American Occupational Therapy Association, 1995). Throughout, *Occupational Therapy* I explain in great detail how the founding generation of occupational therapists divided tasks according to gender as they struggled to attain legitimacy for the new profession.

4. For a discussion of the concept of a therapeutic world view, see T.J. Jackson Lears, *No Place of Grace: Antimodernism and the Transformation of American Culture, 1880–1920* (New York: Pantheon Books, 1981), 47–59.

5. The following studies describe the transformation of women's charity and volunteer work to professional work: LeRoy Ashby, *Saving the Waifs: Reformers and Dependent Children, 1890–1917* (Philadelphia: Temple University Press, 1984); Dorothy G. Becker, "Exit Lady Bountiful: The Volunteer and the Professional Social Worker," *Social Service Review* 34 (March 1964): 57–72; Joan Jacobs Brumberg, "'Ruined' Girls: Changing Community Responses to Illegitimacy in Upstate New York, 1890–1920," *Journal of Social History* 18 (Winter 1984): 247–63; Allen F. Davis, *Spearheads for Reform: The Social Settlement and the Progressive Movement, 1890–1914* (New York: Oxford University Press, 1967); Virginia Drachman, *Hospital With a*

Heart: Women Doctors and the Paradox of Separatism at the New England Hospital, 1862–1969 (Ithaca, N.Y.: Cornell University Press, 1984); Lori D. Ginzberg, *Women and the Work of Benevolence: Morality, Politics, and Class in the Nineteenth Century United States* (New Haven, Conn.: Yale University Press, 1990); Donna L. Franklin, "Mary Richmond and Jane Addams: From Moral Certainty to Rational Inquiry in Social Work Practice," *Social Service Review* 60 (December 1986): 504–25; Nancy A. Hewitt, *Women's Activism and Social Change: Rochester, New York, 1822–1872* (Ithaca, N.Y.: Cornell University Press, 1984); Wendy Kaminer, *Women Volunteering: The Pleasure, Pain, and Politics of Unpaid Work from 1830 to the Present* (Garden City, N.Y.: Anchor Press, 1984); Roy Lubove, *The Professional Altruist: The Emergence of Social Work as a Career, 1880–1930* (Cambridge, Mass.: Harvard University Press, 1965); Robyn Muncy, *Creating a Female Dominion in American Reform, 1890–1935* (New York: Oxford University Press, 1991); Peggy Pascoe, *Relations of Rescue: The Search for Female Moral Authority in the American West 1874–1939* (New York: Oxford University Press, 1990); Julia B. Rauch, "Women in Social Work: Friendly Visitors in Philadelphia, 1880," *Social Service Review* 49 (June 1975): 241–59; and Kathleen Woodroofe, *From Charity to Social Work in England and the United States* (Toronto, Canada: University of Toronto Press, 1962).

6. Katherine Kish Sklar, "Hull House in the 1890s: A Community of Women Reformers." *SIGNS* 10 (1985): 658–77. In this article, Sklar discusses the work of Jane Addams, Julia Lathrop, and Florence Kelley, all of whom lived at Hull House in the 1890s. The three women had similar socioeconomic and educational backgrounds, but as Sklar reveals, along with others such as Grace and Edith Abbott and Sophonisba Breckinridge, they also shared a family political tradition. They all came from families that were involved in the reform movements of the 19th century. All had fathers or brothers who were very active in politics, and this socialized them to promote using political solutions for social problems. At least two important founders of the profession of occupational therapy had similar backgrounds of family activism and close male relatives who were active in politics. Eleanor Clarke Slagle's family was involved in New York State reform movements; her brother was a United States Congressman from New York. Likewise, Elizabeth Upham Davis's parents were active women's suffragists; her father was an attorney for a United States Senator from Wisconsin.

7. Eleanor Clarke Slagle's attendance at the Chicago School of Civics and Philanthropy in summer 1911 is recorded in "Alumni Register, Chicago School of Civics and Philanthropy, 1903–1913," Graham Taylor Papers, Newberry Library, Chicago, p. 64 (Hereafter cited as Graham Taylor Papers). Slagle herself reported the year as 1910 in her unpublished resume "Experience of Eleanor Clarke Slagle," 1922, Papers of the American Occupational Therapy Association, Wilma L. West Library, American Occupational Therapy Foundation, Bethesda, Md. (hereafter cited as AOTA Archives). I have used the school's date throughout this article.

8. Robyn Muncy, *Creating a Female Dominion in American Reform, 1890–1935* (New York: Oxford University Press, 1991).

9. Jane Addams, *Twenty Years at Hull House* (1910; reprint, New York: New American Library, 1960), 261.

10. *Hull House Bulletin* 2 (1897): 9.

11. *Hull House Bulletin* 6 (1903–4): 12.

12. First Report of the Labor Museum at Hull House, Jane Addams Papers, (Main Library; Chicago: University of Illinois at Chicago, ca. 1891, microfilm), p. 15.

13. Ibid.

14. Clifford W. Beers, *A Mind That Found Itself: An Autobiography* (New York: Longmans Green and Company, 1908).

15. Barbara Loomis, "Professional Occupational Therapy Education in Chicago, 1908–1920" (Paper presented at the Written History Serninar Sixty–third Annual Meeting of the American Occupational Therapy Association, Portland, Oreg., April 1983).

16. Graham Taylor, letter to B.R. Burroughs (Secretary, Board of Administration, Springfield, Ill.), 11 March 1910, Graham Taylor Papers.

17. Loomis, "Professional Occupational Therapy Education."

18. Eleanor Clarke Slagle left a remarkable professional record through her work with the American Occupational Therapy Association. Finding accurate data about her personal life, however, has been frustrating. Some information about her early years appears in Edward T. James, Janet W. James, and Paul S. Boyer, eds., *Notable American Women 1607–1950*, vol. 3 (Cambridge, Mass.: Belknap Press of Harvard University Press, 1971), 296–98. The author of the entry describes some of the inconsistencies in the record, even in such basic information as Slagle's correct birth date. For example, Slagle's death record in the New York State Department of Health gives her year of birth as 1876; her tombstone shows the year 1868; and the census records list her age in 1875 as four and in 1880 as nine, which would make her birth year 1871. The 1880 census record for Delhi, First District, contains the following information about the Clark household: "William J. Clark, age 37, ex–sheriff; Emma J. Clark, age 32, wife, keeps house; John D., age 11, son, goes to school; Ella May, age 9, daughter, goes to school; McNett, Belle, servant, age 19; and Murray, John B., boarder, surrogate clerk." No information in any of the sources that I consulted explained when or why Ella May Clark began to use "Eleanor" as her first name and to spell her last name with a terminal "e." Her brother John also changed the spelling of his last name from "Clark" to "Clarke."

19. That there was a 20-year difference in age between William and Emma, or Emmaline, is described in Marian W. Clarke, "Memories of a Congressman's Widow," Marian W. Clarke Papers, New York State Historical Association, Cooperstown, New York. The 1880 census record indicates that there was a 5-year difference in age between them.

20. Paul T. DuVivier, "A Congressman During Hard Times," (Master's thesis, State University of New York at Oneonta, 1976), 1.

21. Ibid., 3.

22. Randall N. Saunders, "Remembering Claverack College" *Hudson Evening Register,* 1944, p. 5. Information about Claverack College is taken from Saunders, "Remembering Claverack College" and "Annual Circular of Claverack College and Hudson River Institute, Claverack, Columbia County, New York," 1881, 1885, 1886, Claverack College Collection, Columbia County Museum, Kinderhook, New York. Ella May Clark is listed in the 1885 and 1886 circulars. Thanks to Helen M. McLallen, curator of the Columbia County Museum, for this information.

23. *The Delaware Gazette* (Cooperstown, N.Y.: New York State Historical Association, 25 April 1894, microfilm).

24. "Slagle, Eleanor Clarke (Mrs.)," ca. 1937, John Davenport Clarke Papers, New York State Historical Association, Cooperstown, New York; James et al., *Notable American Women*, 3:296–98. Slagle's grandniece, Catherine Clarke Colby of Newcastle,

Maine, said in the interview for *Notable American Women,* "There were whole periods of her life she never mentioned," p. 296.

25. Slagle's early career is well described in, "Experience of Eleanor Clarke Slagle."

26. New York Census, Special schedules for Union Veterans of Civil War, (Cooperstown, N.Y.: New York State Historical Association, 1890, microfilm).

27. DuVivier, "A Congressman," 1.

28. Eleanor Clarke Slagle, *State of New York Department of Mental Hygiene, Syllabus for Training of Nurses in Occupational Therapy,* 2nd ed. (New York, 1944), 33.

29. Graham Taylor, letter to Julia Lathrop, 24 November 1913, Graham Taylor Papers.

30. Slagle, "Experience of Eleanor Clarke Slagle,"

31. John Favill, *Henry Bard Favill 1860–1916: A Memorial Volume* (Chicago: Privately Printed, 1917), 13; *History of Medicine and Surgery and Physicians and Surgeons in Chicago* (Chicago: Biographical Publishing Corporation, 1922), 175–76.

32. "Educational Museum: Special Exhibit of Occupations for Invalids" (History of Nursing Collection, Milbank Memorial Library, Columbia University, 16 May to 10 June 1910, mocrofiche), 2374 (hereafter cited as HNC). Herein was mentioned that papers were presented by James E. Russell (Dean of Teachers College), Susan E. Tracy (Superintendent of Nursing at the Adams Nervine Asylum), Mary Lawson Neff (Long Island State Hospital), Herbert J. Hall (Director of the Devereux Workshops in Marblehead, Massachusetts), Livingston Farrand (National Tuberculosis Association), and Arthur Dow (Professor at Teachers College), and later were published in *Proceedings of the American Society of Superintendents of Training Schools for Nursing* (American Society of Superintendents of Training Schools for Nursing, 1910), 172–206.

33. Biographical material on Susan Tracy can be found in Mary Barrows, "Susan E. Tracy, R.N.," *Maryland Psychiatric Quarterly* 6, no. 3 (1917):53–62; Martin Kaufman et al., eds., *Dictionary of American Nursing Biography* (New York and Westport, Conn.: Greenwood Press, 1988), 370–71; Sidney Licht, "The Founding and Founders of the American Occupational Therapy Association," *The American Journal of Occupational Therapy,* 21 (1967): 269–77; Kathryn L. Reed and Sharon R. Sanderson, *Concepts of Occupational Therapy* (Boston, Mass.: Williams and Wilkins Company, 1983), 196–97. According to these sources, Susan E. Tracy is the daughter of Cyrus M. Tracy and Caroline M. (Needham) Tracy; she never married; and she died in 1928 at the age of 50, in the same city in which she was born.

34. Susan E. Tracy, *Studies in Invalid Occupation* (Boston, Mass.: Whitcomb and Barrows, 1910).

35. See Licht, "The Founding," 275; Barrows, "Susan E. Tracy, R. N.," 51–67.

36. Susan C. Johnson, "The Teacher in Occupational Therapy" (Proceedings of the First Annual Meeting of NSPOT, Towson, Md., 1918), 50.

37. Susan E. Tracy, introduction by Daniel H. Fuller, "The Need of Instruction for Nurses in Occupations for the Sick," in *Studies in Invalid Occupation,* (Boston, Mass.: Whitcomb and Barrows, 1910), 3.

38. George M. Beard, *A Practical Treatise on Nervous Exhaustion (Neurasthenia), Its Symptoms, Nature, Sequences, Treatment,* 2nd ed. rev. (New York: W. Wood and Company, 1880), 11–85.

39. Adolph Meyer, "The Philosophy of Occupational Therapy," *Archives of Occupational Therapy*, 1 (1922):1–10. For a discussion of Meyer's career, see Gerald M. Grob, *Mental Illness and American Society 1875–1940* (Princeton, N.J.: Princeton University Press, 1983), 112–118.

40. Fuller, "The Need of Instruction," 4–5.

41. *Thirtieth Annual Report of the Adams Nervine Asylum*, 11.

42. Fuller, "The Need of Instruction," 4–5.

43. Sarah E. Parsons, "Miss Tracy's Work in General Hospitals," *Maryland Psychiatric Quarterly* 6, no. 3 (1917): 63.

44. Barrows, "Susan E. Tracy, R.N.," 53.

45. Fuller, "The Need of Instruction," 4–5.

46. Tracy, *Studies*, 16.

47. Course Descriptions, (HNC; ca. 1911, microfiche), 2374.

48. For an interesting discussion of private–duty nursing and its problems, see Susan M. Reverby, *Ordered to Care: The Dilemma of American Nursing, 1850–1945* (Cambridge, Mass.: Cambridge University Press, 1987), 95–105.

49. William Rush Dunton Jr., "Editorial," *Maryland Psychiatric Quarterly* 6, no. 3 (1917): 52.

50. Reba G. Cameron, "An Interview with Miss Tracy," *Maryland Psychiatric Quarterly* 6, no. 3 (1917), 65.

51. Reverby, *Ordered to Care*, 121–42.

52. Jane Addams, *Twenty Years at Hull House*, 60–71.

53. Lillian Wald, *The House on Henry Street* (New York: Henry Holt and Company, 1915), 1–25.

54. Illinois State Department of Public Welfare, "Founder of Occupational Therapy Work in Illinois," *Welfare Bulletin* (June 1930): 2.

55. Barrows, "Susan E. Tracy, R.N.," 53–61.

56. Barrows, "Susan E. Tracy, R.N.," 59–61.

57. Susan E. Tracy, "The Training of the Nurse as Instructor in Invalid Occupations," in *Proceedings of the American Society of Superintendents of Training Schools for Nurses*, 181–182.

58. Susan E. Tracy, "Report of Classes in Invalid Occupation" (HNC; n.d., microfiche), 2374.

59. Licht, "The Founding," 275.

60. For example, "Report of Committee on Teaching Methods," in *Proceedings of the First Annual Meeting of the National Society for the Promotion of Occupational Therapy* (Towson, Md.: NSPOT, 1917), 34; Susan E. Tracy, "The Influence of Hospital Architecture on Methods of occupational Teaching," in *Proceedings of the First Annual Meeting of National Society for the Promotion of Occupational Therapy* (Towson, Md.: NSPOT, 1917), 42–44; "Report of the committee on Methods," in *Proceedings of the Second Annual Meeting of the National Society for the Promotion of Occupational Therapy* (Towson, Md.: NSPOT, 1918), 20–25.

61. For a discussion of the relationship between the reconstruction movement and occupational therapy, see: Quiroga, *Occupational Therapy*, 115–99.

62. Norma Howat, "Annual Meetings of the Occupational Therapy Profession, 1917–1929," AOTA Archives.

63. Remarks by Dr. W. R. Dunton Jr., "Monday Afternoon Sessions," in *Proceedings of the Third Annual Meeting of the National Society for the Promotion of Occupational Therapy* (Towson, Md.: NSPOT, 1919), 41.

64. "Side Remarks by President Slagle," in *Proceedings of the Fourth Annual Meeting of the National Society for the Promotion of Occupational Therapy* (Towson, Md.: NSPOT, 1920), 4.

65. Howat, "Annual Meetings"; and "President's Report," in *Proceedings of the Fourth Annual Meeting of the National Society for the Promotion of Occupational Theory,* Towson, Md.: NSPOT, 1920), 3; Myra L. McDaniel, "Forerunners of the American Journal of the Occupational Therapy," *American Journal of Occupational Therapy* 25 (1971): 41–52.

66. Since at least 1917, Susan Cox Johnson had believed that a physician ought to lead the association. In a letter to William R. Dunton dated 9 August 1917, she wrote, " I think you should become president of the society because I think we should have a physician in that position," AOTA Archives. Details of the election can be found in "Monday, Morning Session," in *Proceedings of the Third Annual Meeting of National Society of Occupational Therapy* (Towson, Md.: NSPOT, 1919), 35–36.

67. Slagle, "Experience of Eleanor."

68. Remarks by Miss Addams, "Monday Afternoon Session" in *Proceedings of the Third Annual Meeting of the National Society for the Promotion of Occupational Therapy* (Towson, Md.: NSPOT, 1919), 39–41.

69. "Presidents of the American Occupational Therapy Association (1917–1967)," *American Journal of Occupational Therapy* 21 (1967), 290–91.

70. Mrs. Hewitt, "Address of Welcome," in *Proceedings of the Fourth Annual Meeting of the National Society of Occupational Therapy* (Towson, Md.: NSPOT, 1920), 32–33.

71. "The Fifth Annual Meeting of the National Society for the Promotion of Occupational Therapy," 1922, Archives of Occupational Therapy 1, p. 81 (hereafter cited as AOT.

72. Ibid., 82.

73. "The Sixth Annual Meeting of the American Occupational Therapy Association," September 1922, AOT, vol. 2, pp. 81.

74. "Meeting of the Board and Members of the House of Delegates of the American Occupational Therapy Association," 1923, AOT, vol. 2, pp. 53–56.

75. Quiroga, *Occupational Therapy*, 235–38.

76. For a discussion of the postwar reconstruction aides, see Quiroga, "Professional Culture and Education in Occupational Therapy in the 1920s," Stabilization and Standardization in the 1920s, pt. 3, *Occupational Therapy*, 211–32.

77. Ibid., and Men, Medical Identity and Survival in the 1920s, 235–55.

Nursing Reorganization
in Occupied Japan, 1945–1951

Reiko Shimazaki Ryder
Kawasaki University

Although formal nursing education in Japan began as early as 1885, the social, economic, and cultural climate of the country prevented the development of effective training institutions and curricula until 1945 when the American occupation forces directed and supervised the establishment of the present system of nursing education and services. The Americans completely eradicated the previous system, which had been implemented by the Meiji government after the overthrow of the feudal system in 1868. Although the reorganization of nursing and, indeed, the reorganization of Japan in general was nominally carried out through the existing Japanese government, the Japanese people had virtually no power to affect their own national affairs. Reforms were carried out by edict of the American occupation forces with little or no explanation provided to the public.

In July 1948 a new Japanese system for nursing service and education was founded under the supervision of the American occupation forces, largely by means of the Public Health Nurse, Midwife, and Nurse Law 203. Today, we are confronting several problems stemming from the reorganization carried out by the occupation forces, problems not anticipated by either the American or Japanese nurses. Two fundamental problems in nursing can be traced to this foundation. First, most nursing schools are still just certificate programs and are not in the mainstream of higher education. Although Japanese nurses have been trying to transform certificate programs into university programs, they have not yet been very successful. During the restructuring of the political system, nursing education was placed under the jurisdiction of the Ministry of Health and Welfare, not under the Ministry of Education. This resulted in the development of nursing as a vocation, not a profession. The second problem is that the rigid government structure and bureaucratic systems founded by the

Nursing History Review 8 (2000): 71-93. A publication of the American Association for the History of Nursing. Copyright © 2000 Springer Publishing Company.

American occupation forces tended to hinder the efficient handling of problems. This paper discusses several aspects of the immediate postwar occupation to reveal the context from which these problems emerged. Decision-making processes that might have affected the reorganization of Japan by the occupation forces are identified along with the philosophy of medicine and nursing that became the backbone of Japanese nursing.

Modernization of Japan at the End of the 1800s

In 1854, Japan was forced to open the country by Commander Matthew C. Perry who was sent by President Millard Filmore of the United States. Japan had been isolated from the rest of the world because the *Tokugawa Bakufu* (shogunate) held a policy of *Sakoku* (closed country). After this incident the *Tokugawa Bakufu* lost political power in Japan. The Meiji emperor regained the throne, and the modernization of Japan began.

Japan had primarily employed Chinese medicine for hundreds of years with few exceptions. In 1868 the Japanese government finally announced a policy allowing Japanese doctors to practice western medicine. Many medical schools and affiliated hospitals were established. During that time most of the sick were cared for by the patients' families in the home. Hospital inpatients were mainly welfare recipients doctors and medical students treated for their own experience or on whom they could conduct research. The very sick were also hospitalized, but bedside nursing care was left to the patients' families. Soon, doctors found it difficult to work without assistance and began to train nurses for that purpose. Theory was not emphasized at the schools, and the students were trained by apprenticeship. Between 1885 and 1887, two schools of nursing were established in Japan by Linda Richard and M. E. Read, who were missionary nurses from the United States. The curriculum at these schools was similar to that of the St. Thomas School of Nursing in London. Unfortunately, Japan soon became a militaristic and nationalistic country that banned Christianity. Schools sponsored by the U.S. Board of Christianity soon deteriorated. Later, St. Luke's School of Nursing and the Red Cross School of Nursing were established. They were the two major schools of nursing that maintained the quality of nursing education prior to 1945. In response to the emergence of a large number of schools for nursing operated by the hospitals and the medical schools the Ministry of Home Affairs finally issued in 1915 regulations to maintain the standard of nursing education. The regulations addressed areas such as the following:

Article 1, Section 3. The curricula should include:

anatomy and physiolog]y
nursing foundation
hygiene
communicable diseases
sterilization
first aid
national ethics

Article 1, Section 4. Minimum requirement: eighth grade education

Article 1, Section 5. Training period: 2 years

Article 1, Section 6. Principal subjects should be taught by medical doctors[1]

These regulations were not mandated, so that most medical doctors who had their own practice did not comply. Many doctors hired young girls who had only completed compulsory education (sixth grade) and trained them as nurses while they worked as housemaids in their homes. In 1945 this loosely designed nursing education presented a serious obstacle for the American nurses who were eager to raise the standard of nursing service in Japan to the level of American nursing.

Fall of the Japanese Empire

Since the reorganization of nursing was carried out as an integral part of the entire restructuring of Japan's political and social system, it is necessary to understand the way in which the occupation was carried out by the foreign powers. Even before Japan surrendered to the Allied Forces, the United States of America had a plan in place to take total control over the occupation of Japan rather than share joint control with the other Allied powers.[2] Even though the Far Eastern Advisory Commission (a multinational commission) was formed within General Headquarters, Supreme Commander of Allied Powers (GHQ SCAP) to help formulate further policy in Japan, General Douglas MacArthur, as the supreme commander, had complete authority over Japan. The following statement, prepared by the Departments of State and War and the Navy Coordination Committee, and approved by President Harry Truman, was sent to MacArthur to clarify his position in Japan. Dated 6 September 1945, it read as follows:

The authority of the Emperor and the Japanese government to rule the State is subordinate to you as Supreme Commander of the Allied Powers. You will exercise your authority as you deem proper to carry out your mission. Our relations with Japan do not rest on a contractual basis, but on an unconditional surrender. Since your authority is supreme, you will not entertain any question on the part of the Japanese as to its scope.

Control of Japan shall be exercised through the Japanese government to the extent that such an arrangement produces satisfactory results. This does not prejudice your right to act directly if required. You may enforce the orders issued you by the employment of such measures as you deem necessary, including the use of force.[3]

These are the two crucial policies by the occupation forces. First, MacArthur's supremacy meant that the occupation was to be effectively implemented solely by the United States, a single occupation. Second, the use of the existing Japanese government could be used to carry out day-to-day operations, indirect occupation.

MacArthur was a diligent scholar of Japanese history and felt that he had a thorough knowledge of Japanese government, institutions, and culture.[4] He argued that Japan had failed to develop toward the enlightened and progressively minded nation that Perry believed possible in 1854. On 2 September 1945, after the Allied delegates had signed the documents of surrender with Japan aboard the SS *Missouri*, General MacArthur sent a proud and poetic message to the American people. In this message he said:

We stand in Tokyo today reminiscent of our countryman, Commodore Perry, ninety-two years ago. His purpose was to bring to Japan an era of enlightenment and progress by lifting the veil of isolation to the friendship, trade, and commerce of the world. But alas, the knowledge thereby gained of Western science was forged into an instrument of oppression and human enslavement. Freedom of expression, freedom of action, even freedom of thought were denied through suppression of liberal education, through appeal to superstition and through the application of force . . .[5]

With such a historical perspective, MacArthur believed he knew exactly what to do with Japan's reconstruction as a new nation. Put simply, the goal of the occupation was the demilitarization and democratization of Japan.

One of the factors that contributed to the quick recovery of Japan was the adoption of the policy of indirect occupation. Because of the sudden defeat of Japan, the United States' original plan to abolish the entire Japanese government and rule by direct occupation had to be modified to use the existing Japanese bureaucratic system.[6]

As soon as the emperor announced unconditional surrender on 15 August 1945, the Suzuki Cabinet, a military-oriented government, resigned and Prince Higashikuni was appointed as the head of the new government, one of whose policies was protection of the supremacy of the imperial system in Japan.[7] Joseph Grew, Edwin Reischauer, and others who were authorities on Japanese affairs advised the American government to allow Japan to keep the imperial system.[8] *Dilemma in Japan*, written by Andrew Roth in 1945 and widely read by occupation authorities, also suggested the retention of the Emperor but with a reduction of his power and influence on the system of government.[9] The GHQ's plan for the emperor was to make him the symbolic rather than the ruling head of the state.

Centralization of the Bureaucratic System

Japan is a small, compact, and culturally homogeneous country and is therefore relatively easy to govern. Government policies and orders, if well planned and organized, can easily reach every corner of the country. In the beginning of the occupation the GHQ SCAP intended to decentralize the power of the militaristic government. Because of the complete destruction of the country by air raids, the Japanese economy was at its lowest, and the American plan for decentralization could not be accomplished. Because of the limited revenues available to the local government, they could not finance civil agencies such as the fire departments, hospitals, and schools.[10]

Psychological and cultural factors also contributed to the failure of decentralization. From the Meiji era to the end of the war in 1945, Japanese education emphasized the concept of unity and the adherence to national ideology, so that the Japanese people were used to regimentation. Therefore, the Japanese were more comfortable in following orders than in giving them or in making decisions by themselves. Acquiring greater individual rights also made them uncomfortable because they were unsure of how to exert them. Centralization appeared to be better suited to the needs of Japanese society at the time of surrender.

The Military Government Established in Tokyo

MacArthur established the Supreme Command of Allied Powers in Tokyo on 3 October 1945 (Figure 1). GHQ's special staff sections were organized to

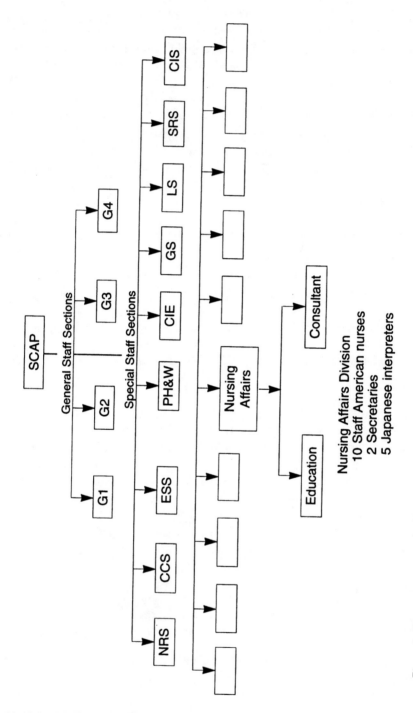

Figure 1. Supreme command of Alice Powers (ACAP).

parallel the functions of the various ministries of the Japanese government. Therefore, each staff section could direct and supervise the respective ministry for which that section was responsible. For instance, the Public Health & Welfare (PH&W) Section was mainly responsible for the Ministry of Health and Welfare of the Japanese government. However, Brigadier General Crawford F. Sams, chief of the PH&W Section (Figure 2), used other staff sections and related ministries of the Japanese government whenever it was required by the nature of the problems.[11]

As for the line of communication from SCAP to the local governments, a centralized system was adopted. Under the central government each prefecture and municipal office was a miniaturized structure of the central government. When SCAP issued a directive, for example, a PH&W Section directive, the Ministry of Health and Welfare was contacted through the Liaison Office; in turn, the Japanese government issued the Imperial Ordinance of Regulation in implementing the directive from GHQ SCAP and sent it to the Medical Affairs Division of the prefectural governments. Thereafter, each prefectural government sent the ordinance to the local medical officials to execute that order.[12]

To ensure compliance by the Japanese government with SCAP's directives, a copy of every ordinance or regulation was sent to the Eighth Army in

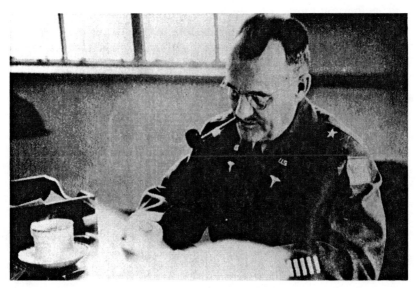

Figure 2. Brigadier General Crawford F. Sams, Chief of the General Headquarters (GHQ) and Public Health & Welfare (PH&W) Section.

Yokohama, which functioned as an operation unit; then a copy was forwarded to the regional military governments located in Hokkaido, Tohoku, Hokuriku, Kinki, Chugoku, Shikoku, and Kyushu. From there each military government would send the ordinance to the military government teams at the prefectural level, whose responsibility was to investigate whether or not the ordinance was being carried out (Figure 3). This system of centralization accelerated the reorganization of Japan. Even after completion of the occupation, the centralization has been maintained to the present. However, the system is no longer entirely functional as it does not meet the needs of a rapidly changing society of this age.

Appointment of the Head of the GHQ PH&W Section

Plans to occupy Japan began at the State Department in Washington, D.C., as early as 1942, while Japan was still scoring spectacular military victories in the Pacific.[13] General John Hilldring was Chief of the Civil Affairs Division in the War Department and a friend of General Sams. When personnel planning for the military government began in early 1945, Hilldring contacted Sams and offered him a position as Chief of the Health, Education and Welfare Division of the military government for the Far East Command.[14]

Because of the heavy casualties suffered by the Japanese army, the Japanese government made a decision to surrender in August of 1945. In the meantime, Sams was interviewing potential staff members for his division. He selected Captain Grace Alt (later Major), a 1933 graduate of the Johns Hopkins School of Nursing with a Bachelor of Science degree from George Peabody College in Nashville, Tennessee (Figure 4).[15] To Sams, Alt appeared to be well qualified because of her prewar teaching experience at a Methodist Missionary Hospital in Korea. That work experience, he believed, would enable her to work with and communicate with Japanese nurses and medical professionals.[16] Because of her past experience, Alt was able to get along well with the Japanese nurses. She was respected and admired for her leadership and understanding of the Japanese people.

Public Health & Welfare Section

Upon Sams' arrival in Yokohama his first assignment was to investigate whether communicable diseases would pose a threat to the American troops

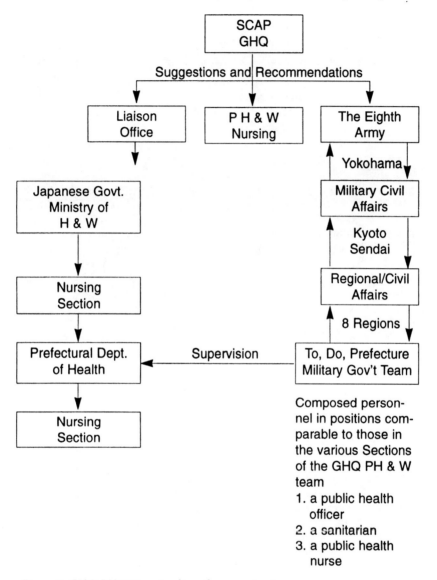

Figure 3. GHQ PH&W section line of communication.

when they landed in Japan. Thus, he set out to investigate health problems in the country. Even though he had some ideas as to what conditions in Japan would be like, Sams was overwhelmed by the devastation caused by the war. As he realized the seriousness and importance of his assignment as Chief of the Health, Education, and Welfare Division, he decided to separate education from his responsibilities. He states:

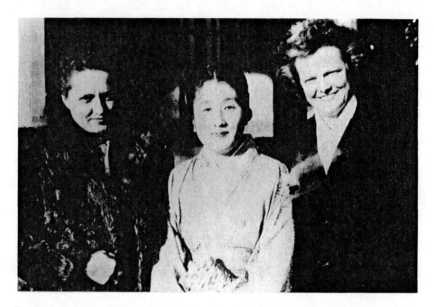

Figure 4. GHQ PH&W around 1945—1951. Left is Major Grace E. Alt, First Chief of the Nurses Division PH&W Section; center is Princess Chichibu; and right is Miss Virginia Olson.

As a Chief of the Health, Education, and Welfare Division of the Military Government Section of the old GHQ, I would have been concerned with both the Ministry of Health and Welfare and the Ministry of Education of the Japanese Government. In studying the problems in these fields with which we were faced after our arrival in Japan in the light of our directives and missions, I came to the conclusion that the task of reorganizing a totalitarian national system of educa-tion, including all elementary and middle (high) schools and universities and technical schools into a decentralized reasonably democratic system, would require the full time and effort of a most capable chief. Likewise the task in the field of Health and Welfare which included the major fields of preventive medicine, medical care, welfare, and social security, was so tremendous that it would also require the best efforts of a single chief.[17]

That decision led to the establishment of two sections, the PH&W Section and the Civil Information and Education Section (later referred to as CI&E). Sams, however, retained his original responsibility for educating health-related professionals, such as medical doctors, dentists, and nurses. He later explained that with nursing schools being affiliated with hospitals at that time he felt confident in his ability to organize more effectively the schools of nursing and nursing management at the hospitals.[18]

Sams had an interesting and colorful background, successfully combining medicine with a military career. His self-assuredness and directness sometimes created conflict and wrong impressions in the minds of the Japanese medical doctors. However, he was very supportive of the Japanese nurses, and his directness helped Japanese nurses to move toward professional autonomy in the patriarchal society of Japan. Sams' philosophy of medicine was to treat a patient as an individual, that is, as a whole person.[19] While serving in the Middle East from 1941 to 1943, he had opportunities to observe the medical system used in British military hospitals in the region. He was disturbed by the overspecialization of medicine practiced in British hospitals.[20] Even though the United States took leadership in the occupation of Japan, multinational troops were stationed in the country, such as from Britain, Australia, France, and the Union of Soviet Socialist Republic (USSR). However, Sams appointed only American nurses to positions in the PH&W Section, Nursing Affairs Division.

He was well aware of the concept of patient-centered nursing care that prevailed in the United States. His philosophy of "total patient care" had the full support and agreement of the staff in the Nursing Affairs Division. Since Sams completely trusted Alt to reorganize the Japanese nursing system he endowed her with complete authority to direct the reform. Alt and the other nursing staff members' first task was to teach Japanese nurses their philosophy of nursing. Alt had expressed her view of nursing in the foreword to the *Nursing Procedure Manual*, published by the Medical Friend *Sha* (company) in 1947. She wrote:

> Nursing has been and will be a profession that was born from the spirit of benevolence. Nursing is art, science, and a profession as well. Nursing is creative, dramatic, and it can never separate from human living.[21]

Japanese nursing reform was then carried out on the basis of this nursing philosophy; that is, "Nursing is art, science, and a profession."

One of the reasons why nursing reform in Japan was so successful was that Alt had a pleasant personality and was skillful in dealing with the Japanese.[22] She used human resources intelligently, especially the graduates from St. Luke's School of Nursing, Tokyo, who could speak English fluently. One of them was Mitsu Kaneko, who often accompanied the GHQ nurses on inspection trips. Kaneko was called to the GHQ almost every day, along with Natsue Inoue, Masu Yumaki, and Masae Hirai, to discuss how to carry out reforms in Japanese nursing.[23]

Establishment of the Nursing Education Council

After preliminary investigation of the existing schools of nursing and hospital services, Alt formed the Nursing Education Council on 25 March 1946. Even though the name of the council implied "nurses," the membership consisted of Japanese medical doctors and officials of the Japanese government so that reorganization in nursing would be carried out more effectively. At this council they discussed matters such as the establishment of model schools, new nursing laws, refresher courses for existing nurses, and innovations in nursing services at the hospitals.

The Nursing Education Council assessed the nursing reports presented by the Nursing Affairs Division and reached the conclusion that a new nursing law should be promulgated. In the meantime, in June 1946 the Tokyo Model Demonstration School of Nursing (later referred to as the Tokyo Model School of Nursing) was established for the purpose of experimenting with the new curriculum discussed in the Nursing Education Council and establishing a paradigm for other new nursing schools to follow (Figure 5). The foundation of the Tokyo Model School of Nursing was laid immediately after the

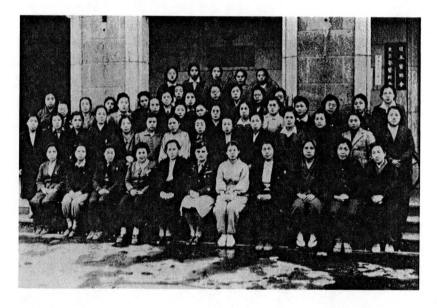

Figure 5. Captain (later Major) Grace E. Alt, A. N. C., and Japanese midwifery leaders in conference.

occupation began. As soon as Sams arrived in Japan in August 1945, he began to search for potential hospitals which might be converted into an American army hospital. He loved St. Luke's Hospital at first sight and decided to confiscate it immediately. As a result, one of the most prestigious schools of nursing, St. Luke's College of Nursing, lost the facility in which its students practiced their profession and thus faced the crisis of having to discontinue its program. Sams thought it would be a good idea to use St. Luke's College of Nursing as a model school of nursing by merging it with another school of nursing until the hospital could be returned to the Episcopalian church organization.[24]

At that time the Red Cross Schools of Nursing were commonly acknowledged by the public as the best schools of nursing because of the widely publicized achievements of their graduates in the Sino-Japanese War, the Russo-Japanese War, World War I, and World War II. Since the Central Red Cross Hospital, which had been used as an army hospital in Tokyo, had miraculously escaped damage from the air raids, the physical facilities and medical equipment were well preserved. Sams proposed merging St. Luke's College of Nursing into the Central Red Cross School of Nursing. Sams' idea materialized when Prince Tokugawa Kuniyuki of the Red Cross Society and Dr. Hirotosi Hashimoto of St. Luke's College of Nursing signed a contract on 30 April 1946. On 1 June 1946, students from St. Luke's College of Nursing and the Central Red Cross School of Nursing were merged into one student body. From that time on the faculty of both institutions made great efforts to make the merger successful by resolving their differences.

In the beginning, American nurses participated in teaching, but gradually, Japanese faculty, especially those from St. Luke's, assumed leadership in teaching students the theories and fundamentals of nursing. Mary Collins, nursing education consultant of the Nursing Affairs Division, believed that merely acquiring a knowledge of medicine and nursing was not sufficient for providing good patient care. She said:

> The art of nursing is acquired only by doing. Therefore, learning nursing art is only accomplished by actual participation in real situations by the bedside . . . without a theoretical foundation the student nurses can not apply theory into practice.[25]

In light of this, American nurses spent much of their time in the hospital units and concentrated their efforts on internal reorganization of nursing service, physical settings, and even improving the doctors' attitudes toward nurses. They left nursing education mainly in the hands of Japanese faculty members. Besides this model school, PH&W Section, GHQ, encouraged the establishment of similar schools of nursing in each prefecture. Such schools played important ro!es in disseminating the new philosophy of nursing and in raising the quality of nursing education.

Formation of Nursing Law 203

Soon after the occupation began, Alt gave a speech at the Central Red Cross Hospital in Tokyo in which she stated that the goal of the reorganization of nursing by the occupation forces was to strive to improve the quality of nurses and nursing service. She further stated that the entrance qualification for the school of nursing would be raised and that the existing curriculum would be revised and expanded, making it more appropriate for meeting professional needs.[26] In order to improve and implement standards of nursing, there had to be an independent nursing law. As noted earlier, there had been a nursing law, promulgated in 1915, but it never was effectively implemented. During the war, nursing regulations were included in the National Medical Treatment Law of 1942, which also covered doctors, dentists, and pharmacists. On 11 April 1946, Alt instructed the members of the Nursing Education Council to review the curricula of American nursing schools and propose a new curriculum for the Japanese. Eventually, the Public Health Nurse, Midwife and Nurse Law 203 was promulgated on 3 July 1948. The purpose of the new law and the definition of nurses were stipulated in the law.

Article I. This law shall aim to elevate the quality of the public health nurse, midwife, and nurse, and then, to attempt popularization and elevation of medical treatment and public health.

Article II. In this law, "public health nurse" shall mean a female who has been licensed by the Ministry of Welfare and practices guidance with respect to health under the title of public health nurse.

Article III. In the law, "midwife" shall mean the female who has been licensed by the Minister of Welfare and practices midwifery or guidance with respect to the health of pregnant women, women in childbed and newly born babies.

Article IV. The nurse shall be class-A nurses and class-B nurses.

Article V. In this law, "class-A nurses" shall mean the female who has been licensed by the Minister of Welfare and practices nursing for the injured, the sick, or women in childbed or assistance for medical examination and treatment.

Article VI. In this law, "class-B nurses" shall mean the female who has been licensed by a prefectural governor and practices the practice mentioned in the preceding Article (except nursing for the injured, the sick or women in childbed who are acute and heavy) under the direction of a medical practitioner, a dentist, or a class-A nurse.[27]

Hirai, Inoue, and others wished for the reorganization of nurses into a single category of clinical nurse, but Collins persuaded them to establish two levels, which resulted in the creation of class-A and class-B nurses.[28] A class-A nurse, a graduate from senior high school, had to pass a national examination after graduating from a 3-year accredited school of nursing, while a class-B nurse, a junior high school graduate, needed to pass a prefectural nursing examination after completing the course of study of a 2-year accredited school of nursing. A midwife or public health nurse had to complete 1 year of education specifically tailored to her specialty after 3 years of basic training as a clinical nurse.

Those who wished to organize nursing as a single category of clinical nurses were probably eager to raise nursing standards but failed to appreciate the real situation facing Japan. Nurses were urgently needed by the hospitals, where numerous patients were suffering and dying from starvation and communicable diseases. Nurses were needed by the public health centers to teach disease prevention and to promote health. Class-B nurses could be helpful in reducing the shortage of nurses. Sams explained why it was necessary to train class-B nurses. He said that during the 1940s the concept of nursing teams had been studied in the United States.[29] As a matter of fact, Eleanor Lamberstson was developing the theory of team nursing at Teachers College, Columbia University. According to this theory, nurse's aids and practical nurses could work minor jobs according to their abilities so that registered nurses could devote themselves to their own unique functions.

Supplementary Courses for Existing Nurses

The members of the Nursing Education Council unanimously agreed to provide supplementary courses for existing nurses to prepare them for the national examination. Dr. Y. Nishimori, a member of the Nursing Education Council from Jikei-kai Medical College, told the members of the council that the existing nurses needed more science courses because, not having gone through high school, they were very weak in the fundamentals of chemistry, physics, and so on. He suggested providing these courses. However, Collins countered that applicants for the refresher courses had passed entrance examinations in those subjects. Additionally, Ko Kuge, who was an officer of the Ministry of Health, suggested that nurses, whether they were applying for the national nurses' examination or not, had to be given the opportunity to take refresher courses so that they could learn more about their profession. Whether doctors or nurses, all were obligated to take refresher courses at certain times. However, mandatory education was not implemented because the concept seemed too impractical. The Nursing Education Council meeting resulted in implementing systematic supplementary courses throughout Japan after 1947. These courses were given at the national, regional, prefectural, and hospital in-service education levels. There was a pattern common to all the supplementary courses, whether national, regional, or prefectural, although there were variations in the content and order of subjects offered. In 1947, Alt assigned Billie Harter to set up a series of refresher courses for fifty potential teachers sent by forty-six prefectures. The purpose of the program was to teach the new philosophy of nursing—to teach patient-centered care—for which a basic knowledge of science was required of the nurses to insure safe care of the patient. Harter said:

> We were diligently teaching new ideas and principles to very young students in the basic nursing program, but it would be a very long time before they could work in positions of authority and leadership in the existing hospital situation. There needed to be older teachers who had a similar education who could go back to their hospitals throughout Japan with an understanding of the philosophy and some knowledge of application and most of all enthusiasm for implementing the new idea in their hospitals.[30]

The curriculum included anatomy, physiology, microbiology, medical-surgical nursing, basic nursing procedures, communicable diseases, and principles of teaching. The PH&W Section reported that a total of 3,524 nurses had received certificates of completion for the courses given by the various organizations during the intense period of the Japanese occupation. More than 14,000 nurses received training under these programs.[31] The success of nursing reorganization may be truly attributed to the extensive education that disseminated the knowledge and skills of nursing to the nurses in peripheral areas through in-service, prefectural, regional, and national programs. This system of providing refresher courses is still being implemented by the Japanese Nurses Association.

Reorganization of a Professional Organization

At the time of surrender, Japan had three separate nursing organizations: the *sanba* (midwife) organization, nurses organization, and public health nurses organization. The *sanba* organization was the most powerful and active of all. By the end of the war, there were 62,209 midwives of whom only 5,753 had completed the midwifery courses. In 1943, 96.3% of all deliveries were reported to have been carried out by midwives. The president of the *sanba* organization was either a medical doctor or a politician. During the first phase of the occupation, GHQ SCAP purged the war criminals, collaborators, and high-ranking medical doctors in the military services. Alt believed that the *sanba* organization should be dissolved in order to eliminate the taint of militarism and nationalism and also because with the organization being run by medical doctors, nurses did not have the power of decision making within their own organization.

At a Nursing Education Council meeting in April 1946, GHQ nurses presented the constitution and bylaws of the American Nurses Association as a model and suggested the founding of a single unified organization to be called the Midwife, Public Health Nurse and Nurse Association (later renamed the Japanese Nurses Association). On 22 November 1946, after more than 6 months of discussion, a national meeting was held to discuss the establishment of this association. Arriving at a consensus in the meeting was not easy because some nurses, especially the midwives, opposed the unified association. Finally, Inoue, who was serving as chair, told the audience, acting on Collins' advice, to remain in their seats if they agreed to the proposed constitution and bylaws of the national organization and to leave the auditorium if they disagreed. She said to the audience, " We would like to go ahead with the plan even if the membership is small." The auditorium became quiet; nobody left. Without hesitation, Inoue declared consensus.[32] Between 1947 and 1953 all forty-six prefectures had branches of the Japanese Nurses Association that were very active in providing educational programs and in improving nursing services in the hospitals.

Innovation of Hospital Administration and Services

To the American nurses, nursing service and nursing education were insepa-rable. Therefore, reorganization was always conducted with both components in mind. Most Japanese hospitals, however, were organized to accommodate

the needs of medical education and were rigidly departmentalized and bureaucratic. The GHQ had to break up this traditional structure in order to
democratize the health care system. Each department of a hospital had a special
function or specialty and was headed by a chief medical doctor who had a
complete unit, including an X-ray room, laboratory, and so on, at his disposal.
The chief had his own staff: assistant professors, lecturers, medical staff, head
nurse, nurses, and a janitor, in that order of importance. Nurses were assigned
to the doctors and did whatever they were ordered to do. The head nurse's
living quarters were in the patients' area, and she stayed there around the clock.
Virginia Ohlson, the Second Chief of the Nursing Affairs Division, described
hospital conditions as follows:

> . . . Nurses once assigned to a department were rarely rotated to other services.
> Their duties consisted of assisting the doctors as necessary, taking temperatures,
> giving medications and some treatments, and keeping the wards and clinics clean.
> When a department chief and his assistants had a schedule in an outpatient clinic
> or surgery, the same nurses who worked on the hospital wards followed to assist
> them, frequently leaving the wards without nursing supervision. There were no
> night duty nurses; nurses who worked during the day slept in adjoining rooms on
> the hospital wards where patients or their family attendants could call them
> during the night if necessary. All nurses took their orders directly from members
> of the medical staff. Each department had a head nurse, but she assumed little or
> no responsibility for the nursing staff but was primarily concerned with helping
> the department chief and his assistants.[33]

When existing schools of nursing applied for reclassification as a new
school of nursing, American nurses of the military government team in that
prefecture summoned a nursing teacher from the school and a nurse from an
affiliated hospital to discuss reclassification procedures. For example, the
Kyushu University School of Nursing, built in the Meiji era, applied for the
new program in 1948. Josephine Barker, an American nurse working in the
Kyusyu District and responsible for implementing directives from the GHQ,
and Sue Nakamura, the head of the nursing department at the Medical Affairs
Division in Fukvoka prefecture and responsible for carrying out directives
under the supervision of Barker, visited the hospital and told the hospital to
eliminate all family members and attendants from the patients' bedside and to
hire nurses aides instead. Barker instructed the hospital director to establish a
more democratic administration organization including a director of nursing,
and also to set up a central kitchen and housekeeping so that nurses could
concentrate on their own work.[34]

At that time, there were 322 attendants or family members staying with
patients at the Kyushu University Hospital. They were all removed from the
floors, and 50 of them were hired as nurses' aides.

In northern Japan, Hokkaido University also applied for the new nursing program. Before the program began, Katsu Yamazaki and Kiyoshi Kasai were sent to Tokyo to take the refresher course for potential teachers. Yamazaki had never experienced such exciting and dynamic classes before, and she returned to her hospital full of hope for the future of nursing. With her new vision and enthusiasm she began to reorganize nursing service at the hospital. She faced countless problems that would interfere with this task, but her persistence and patience along with the American nurses' support made reform possible.[35]

The main problem that confronted her was the doctors' lack of understanding of nursing. For example, doctors complained that their patients frequently caught colds because the nurses gave them bed baths. They rebuked the nurses in front of the patients. Doctors also complained that nurses were wasting much of their time on recording nursing notes. Sams recognized the situation well. He said:

> We had some major problems. One was an attempt to reorient the concept of the Japanese that patient care in the hospital was the responsibility of the patient's family [and] impressing on the hospital director that the feeding and nursing care of the patient was really responsibility of the hospital staff.[36]

A critical part of this reorganization was the establishment of a separate department of food services, housekeeping, and laundry so that nurses could devote their attention to the care of patients. The establishment of nursing departments gave nurses more autonomy in the hospitals. Doctors were no longer in charge of nursing with regard to the nurse's employment, assignment, and nursing activities.

The patients' families who were caring for the patients were removed from the bedside and nurses took full responsibility in caring for those patients. The tasks of scrubbing and cleaning the clinics were delegated to the housekeeping department. Nurses thus gradually became capable of carrying out their own tasks and responsibilities.

Educating the Medical Profession

In September 1948, Sams and his staff gave a short course on hospital administration to hospital directors from all parts of Japan. After completing the courses, medical doctors returned to their hospitals and launched the reforms. At the same time they provided in-service education to the medical staff on the new concept of hospital administration and management. At Hokkaido University Hospital the director told his staff not to address nurses saying "*oi*" (hey) and instructed them not to use nurses for private purposes since the new nurses would be reflecting a higher standard of nursing education. Nurses were no longer to be regarded as their assistants or servants but were to be looked upon as equals, like the wheels of a car.[37]

Conclusion

These reformations were accomplished within 6 years. The nursing reorganization was successfully and efficiently accomplished because changes were made systematically, following the problem-solving approach. Also, the American government had conducted thorough research on Japan's history, culture, institutions, and people. Being familiar with the country as it existed before the occupation enabled the nursing reorganization to be integrated with the reorganization of other social, educational, and medical institutions. The goal to be met and problems to be solved were discussed with Japanese nurses and all others concerned, including doctors and government officials. American nurses showed strong leadership, tempered by the human qualities of compassion, understanding, and fairness. As Japanese nurses were well aware of the need to reorganize the nursing system, they admired the American nurses' leadership and followed their advice and directives faithfully. American nurses never mandated reforms but rather encouraged the Japanese nurses to make use of American authority to break through the rigid Japanese bureaucratic system for the betterment of nursing.

After the occupation had ended the development of Japanese nursing education was very slow in terms of transforming nursing schools into collegiate schools because of the rigid bureaucratic system in Japan. In 1985, there were only eleven collegiate schools of nursing. The Japanese Nurses Association has sent several nurses to the upper diet as representatives of the nursing profession. They have worked for revision of the nursing law to update and to incorporate changes to create a better health care system to meet the needs of the people in the community.

Now, the Japanese public and the Japanese government are both aware of the importance of the nurses' role. Within 10 years, fifty-three collegiate schools of nursing have been established. Today, the Japanese nurses have more confidence and are more assertive in dealing with health problems and nursing affairs. This is a fruitful consequence of the reorganization in the postwar period.

The issues remaining to be addressed in the coming years are political reform, the promotion of decentralization, and the need for each school to construct its own curriculum on the basis of its individual philosophy. Japanese bureaucratic institutions lack flexibility, and are incapable of revising laws and systems once they have been implemented. This must be rectified to comply with the needs of the age. The existing nursing laws of the Ministry of Health and Welfare have undergone many amendments but are insufficient for providing adequate education for nurses in their expanded nursing roles.

Increasing the efficiency of the present institution of nursing cannot happen without fundamental reform of the Public Health Nurse, Midwife, and Nurse Law. We nurses must strive to become intimately involved in political activities to make sure that we are well represented in government legislature by vigorously undertaking lobbying activities and by directing our students— the nurses of the future—to take an active interest in politics.

The postwar reform included the inception of the Nursing Department within the Ministry of Welfare to represent nursing. It is hoped that the significance of this original objective will not be forgotten, allowing for the construction of a better system for nursing. It is essential to maintain a clear vision that goes beyond simply keeping in line with existing laws and regulations, thus aspiring to the overall elevation of medical and nursing care in the nation.

REIKO SHIMAZAKI RYDER, RN, EDD
    Professor
    Kawasaki: University of Medical Welfare
    The Department of Nursing
    Kurashiki-City, Okayama-Ken, #701-0114
    Japan

Acknowledgment

The author acknowledges the guidance and encouragement of Dr. Joan E. Lynaugh and Assistant Professor Toshiko Yamada. Without their assistance, this article would not have been completed. The photographs used here were provided by the U.S. Army Center of Military History, Washington, D.C., and various other sources in Japan.

Notes

1. *Koseishyo Imukyoku Kangoka Kango Roppo* (Tokyo: Shin Nippon Hoki Syuppangaisya, 1979), 596.
2. Jon Livingston, Joe Moore, and Felicia Oldfather, ed., *Postwar Japan 1945 to the Present* (New York: Pantheon Books, 1973), 3.
3. Government Section, Supreme Commander of Allied Powers (SCAP), *Political Reorientation of Japan* (Washington, D.C.: Government Printing Office, n.d.), 427.
4. Masamichi Royama, *Yomigaeru Nippon* (Tokyo: Chuokoronsha, 1967), 37.
5. SCAP, *Political Reorientation*, 737.
6. Eiji Takemae, *Senryo Sengoshi: Tainichi Kanri Seisaku no Zenyo* (Tokyo: Soshisha, 1980), 36–38.
7. Royama, *Yomigaeru Nippon*, 44.
8. Takemae, *Senryo Sengoshi*, 94.
9. Masataka Kosaka, foreword to *A History of Postwar Japan*, by E. O. Reischauer (Tokyo: Kodansha International Ltd., 1972), 37.
10. Crawford F. Sams, n.d., "Medic," box 1, Sams Collection, The Hoover Institution on War, Peace and Revolution, Standford, Calif., p. 388.
11. Crawford F. Sams, interview by author, tape recording, Atherton, Calif., 22 May 1982.
12. Sams, "Medic," 383–94.
13. Ibid.
14. Crawford F. Sams, letter to author, 18 May 1981.
15. Pauline E. Maxwell, *History of the Army Nurse Corps, 1775–1976* (Washington, D.C.: U.S. Army Center of Military History, 1976), 180.
16. Sams, interview.
17. Crawford F. Sams, *Decision-SCAP* (Stanford, Calif.: The Hoover Institution on War, Peace and Revolution, n.d.), 382–83.
18. Crawford F. Sams, letter to author, 25 March 1981.
19. Interview with Sams, 22 May 1982.
20. Crawford F. Sams, letter to author, 22 August 1982.
21. Grace E. Alt, foreword to the *Nursing Procedure Manual* (Tokyo: Medical Friend Sha, 1947), 4.
22. Sams, interview.
23. Masae Hirai, letter to author, 1982
24. Crawford F. Sams, letter to author, 8 August 1980.
25. Mary Collins, "Ward Supervision," *The Japanese Journal of Nursing* (November 1946), 2–4.
26. Grace E. Alt, "Mission of the Red Cross Nurses," in *Hakuai* (Tokyo: Red Cross Society, 1946), 10.
27. Crawford F. Sams, n.d., *The Public Health Nurse, Midwife, and Nurses Law*, box 8, Sams collection, The Hoover Institution on War, Peace, and Revolution, Stanford, Calif., p. 203.
28. Nursing Education Council, Minutes of Meeting, February 1947, General National Archives, Washington, D.C.

29. Crawford F. Sams, letter to author, 20 April 1980.

30. Billie Harter, letter to author, 28 March 1980.

31. "Public Health and Welfare Section, General Headquarters (GHQ), SCAP," in *Public Health and Welfare in Japan, August 1945-July 1948* (n.p., n.d.).

32. Natsue Inoue, *Wagamaeni Michiwa Hiraku* (Tokyo: Japanese Nursing Association, 1978), 110.

33. Virginia Ohlson, "The History of Nursing Education in Japan" (Master's thesis, University of Chicago, 1955) 57–58.

34. Tomoe Sukouchi and Kotomi Tsuru, interview by author, tape recording, Fukuoka Nurses Association, Fukuoka, Japan, 26 November 1982.

35. Katsu Yamazaki, letter to author, 3 March 1982.

36. Sams, "Medic," 528.

37. Yamazaki, letter, 3 March 1982.

Springer Publishing Company

American Nursing
A Biographical Dictionary

New

Vern L. Bullough, RN, PhD and **Lilli Sentz,** MLS

"As far as I know, none of this type of material is yet online in any of the data bases related to nursing history."

-Joan E. Lynaugh, Emeritus Professor and Term Chair,
Center for the Study of the History of Nursing,
University of Pennsylvania School of Nursing

From the frontier to the university, here is an exciting collection of biographies of individual nurses in the United States and Canada since 1925. Everyone knows a few important nurses, such as Lavinia Dock or Adelaide Nutting or Margaret Sanger. Yet there were many more who wrote the books, founded the schools and organizations, and fought the struggles to advance nursing. Information about most of them is difficult to come by for several reasons. Nurses were overwhelmingly female and generally came from the wrong class. They were not listed in the Who's Who of the past, or even in collections like Notable American Women.

This is a list of several hundred names compiled through the help of nurse historians and volunteers from the American Association for the History of Nursing. It gives nurses a real sense of their history which is not available anywhere else. The contributors of the biographies in an act of scholary devotion preserve a sense of the profession's past.

American Nursing: A Biographical Dictionary, Volume Three is an invaluable reference work for students and librarians. Fully illustrated with many one-of-a-kind photographs.

2000 360pp. 0-8261-1296-x *hard* *$69.95 tentative*
www.springerpub.com

536 Broadway, New York, NY 10012-3955 • (212) 431-4370 • Fax (212) 941-7842

Medical Service to Settlers
The Gestation and Establishment of a Nursing Service in Québec, 1932–1943

NICOLE ROUSSEAU
Faculté de sciences infirmières
Université Laval

JOHANNE DAIGLE
Département d'histoire
Université Laval

The depression of the 1930s pushed the government of Québec to give land to indigent persons desirous of settling in Québec's remote regions. This movement created small communities called settlements comprised principally of very poor people. For several reasons, not the least of which were budgetary constraints, the government decided to hire nurses to serve the health care needs of these settlements instead of subsidizing doctors. This choice forced the government to accept the fact that nurses daily did what were essentially considered medical acts. Thus the Medical Service to Settlers (MSS) was created in 1936 to supervise the establishment, financing and administration of nurses' dispensaries.[1] It became a division of the Québec Ministry of Health in 1943 and was abolished in 1962, but its nurses, still viewed as indispensable, were integrated into the County Health Units, and accounts of their activities were included in the annual reports of the Ministry of Social Affairs until 1971. Even then, while descriptions of their activities disappeared from the official reports, the government of Québec continued to maintain and even open new residential dispensaries run by nurses.[2] No less than 174 nursing posts were created by the provincial government since 1932, most under the auspices of the MSS and with a residential dispensary. Using mainly archival data, we have produced a map of the network thus constituted; to give an idea of the isolation

Nursing History Review 8 (2000): 95-116. A publication of the American Association for the History of Nursing. Copyright © 2000 Springer Publishing Company.

of these outposts, suffice it to say that Val-d'Or is 531 km (330 miles) northwest of Montréal and that, still today, the only road on the north shore of the Saint Lawrence River stops at Natashquan.[3] Yet, the extent of the phenomenon and its persistence are not fully recognized in the historiography.[4]

The origins and evolution of a "nursing" service in Québec called "Medical" Service to Settlers raise several questions and cover a period that we have divided into four subperiods: the gestation and the service (1932–1943), its maintenance and the expansion (1944–1961), its decline (1962–1971), and its remains (1972 to today). Here we shall discuss the gestation and establishment of the service over 10 years from 1932 to 1943. What caused the provincial government to implement such a service? Where did the idea come from to establish dispensaries with resident nurses? How did this solution, deemed temporary and set up to serve urgent needs during the Great Depression of the 1930s, come to be maintained during the World War II? We will argue that the government of Québec, involved in a project of colonization, was compelled by circumstances to establish, finance and administer a network of residential dispensaries operated by nurses. We shall show how this service, "the most reasonable solution,"[5] became solidly established despite the reluctance and hesitation of the authorities. We will also offer a glimpse at the vast array of operations performed by the nurses and the heroic conditions in which they worked. The main inspiration comes from an analysis of the MSS archives and from the accounts of the nurses' activities included in the annual reports of the provincial Ministry of Health.[6]

The Gestation of a Necessity-Inspired Solution (1932–1935)

Before the Great Depression of the 1930s, there were a few nurses posted in remote areas that lacked doctors.[7] The work of Father Louis Garnier, Eudist missionary, provides a general idea of the circumstances surrounding the creation of these nursing posts. In his account of the missionaries' experience on the north shore in the early years of the twentieth century, he notes that, in the absence of doctors,

> Almost all [the missionaries] handled medical problems, gave advice and proposed known remedies. Several became experts in pulling teeth. But so many times [he adds] they left the bedrooms of patients perplexed and worried, not knowing what to do nor what to say![8]

In 1922 it would appear that, in the hope of obtaining doctors to serve the more important centers of the region, Garnier contacted Dr. Alphonse Lessard; this physician was simultaneously director of both the Bureau of Public Charities (BPC) and the Provincial Bureau of Health (PBH) from 1921 to 1936.[9] Following the pressure exerted by Garnier, who was posted at Rivière-au-Tonnerre, a small place on the north shore, Lessard ordered a medical inspection of the region; the medical inspection report, filed in 1924, mentions "appalling" hygienic conditions in the 17 municipalities visited between Godbout and Natashquan.[10] In 1926 the director of the PBH authorized the hiring of a nurse; this is the first post for which we possess information. Thus, on 26 August 1926, nurse Eveline Bignell set herself up in a rented house in order to receive and treat anyone who came to her and to perform childbirth and do house calls when needed. Two other nurses were hired in the same way in 1929 to serve Rivière-Saint-Jean and Natashquan, two places on the north shore which lacked medical services.

According to Garnier the idea to have recourse to the services of nurses was due to the high sums asked for by doctors to serve poor areas: "Thus, a problem, formerly a source of anguish, found its most reasonable solution for the North Shore and for poor and isolated areas."[11] In 1932, Lessard saw this solution as "the most reasonable" as well for the new settlements in the province,[12] but as we shall see, it took years before it would be accepted and financed on a regular, if not permanent, basis. The idea faced important obstacles, especially the opposition of doctors, the lack of legislation for financing such services, and the sharing of responsibilities between the PBH and the Ministry of Colonization. It was by introducing the practice as a "temporary solution" that the protagonists of the MSS succeeded in getting the new service accepted.

"THE MOST REASONABLE SOLUTION" TOLERATED ON A TEMPORARY BASIS
In the spring of 1932 the federal government established a land settlement program as a means of helping the unemployed in the cities and the poor farmers. This program, the Gordon Plan, required financial contributions from both the provincial and municipal governments for the settlement of families on the land. The allocation offered ($600) was insufficient, and the government of Québec had to financially support the growing settlements by handing out bonuses for forest clearing, schools, construction, and salaries of civil servants, school teachers and nurses, who were sent to places where needs appeared urgent.[13] Sending nurses instead of doctors, even as a temporary measure, met with a few obstacles at the very beginning. The post finally set up at Auclair, a settlement in the lower Saint Lawrence, illustrates some of the

difficulties encountered in the application of this solution. Lessard wrote about this settlement to the Minister of Colonization in December 1932 that he had "already received complaints from certain doctors who are opposed to the appointment of nurses."[14] The instructions to the nurses indicate the desire of the PBH to minimize the risk of potential conflicts. In January 1933, in the letter of engagement of the nurse for Auclair, Gabrielle Blais, Dr. Émile Nadeau explained the situation and temporary nature of her position; he also insisted that "the Bureau of Public Charities will not be responsible for the fees incurred unless a special agreement is reached in each case. . . ."[15]

The responsibility of the Bureau of Public Charities was limited to covering part of the hospitalization costs of people recognized as indigent, and these did not include doctors' fees.[16] Aside from her salary, no budget had been foreseen to finance the cost of the nurse's services. In the early 1930s a few other nurses were appointed with the same precautions and on a temporary basis in Abitibi-Témiscamingue (Aurore Bégin in 1932 at Rollet, Blanche Esnouf in 1934 at Sainte-Gertrude de Manneville, and Murielle Lemieux in 1935 at Lac Barrière), in the Saguenay (Anita Dionne in 1932 at Anse Saint-Jean), and in the lower Saint Lawrence (Luce Thibault, 1 January 1932, at Biencourt).

Under pressure to go further than these urgent and selective actions and to move in favor of what many people considered a work of restoration,"[17] the liberal government of L. A. Tachereau announced on 8 August 1934 its intention to submit to the legislature a vast colonization plan (which became the Vautrin Plan), conceived and financed entirely by the province, and to invest $10,000,000.[18] On 17 and 18 October 1934, at the Colonization Conference held in Québec, the means of applying the projected plan were discussed. Lessard, as director of the PBH, explained to the three hundred or so persons[19] assembled the measures already taken by his service to assure settlers of certain areas a minimum of medical assistance and again insisted on the extraordinary and temporary nature of these measures:

> We are undergoing a crisis and in extraordinary times one must take extraordinary measures. In a completely temporary manner, we have established at the river Solitaire [Témiscamingue] in the townships of Biencourt and Auclair [Lower St Lawrence], in the township of Villemontel [Abitibi], where there are large numbers of settlers, nurses who give first aid to victims of accidents or to sick patients and who do childbirth. We have instructed them, when a special case arises, to send . . . to hospital . . . patients for whom they are not certain to be able to provide the necessary treatment. Also, we have a doctor who goes constantly from one end of the province to the other. . . . He supervises the work of the nurses. When he passes through settlement areas, he gives consultations. This is what we have done.[20]

The doctor traveling around the province alluded to by Lessard was Dr. Émile Martel, who became regional doctor-hygienist and medical officer of the County Health Unit of the recently established county of Abitibi. The assembly refused, however, to sanction the solution proposed by Lessard, which consisted in appointing "a doctor in a region with a certain number of nurses under his orders"; the director of the PBH had, however, admitted that ". . . in all the settlement areas where we developed the system, the effect has been magnificent."[21] The assembly supported rather the proposition presented by Dr. J. E. Desroches, president of the settlement medical societies, to wit ". . . That the provincial Government, in its settlement program, see to the appointment of doctors in all the new areas where the need shall be felt. . . ."[22] However, none of the laws adopted during the 1930s which touched settlements obliged the provincial government to assure such medical service. Desrochers's resolution would remain a dead letter as we shall see shortly.

Before the special budget allocated to the Ministry of Colonization for the establishment of the Vautrin Plan was voted, Martel, no doubt informed about the above resolution, tried to apply the latter in a particular case. Indeed, in his capacity as medical officer of the County Health Unit of Abitibi, he sent, on 18 February 1935, to the director of the PBH a report in three parts: (1) health inspection, (2) education in hygiene, and (3) medical aid to settlers. In this last part, he proposed to Lessard the trial, in the Duparquet area of Abitibi, a system of medical aid to settlers that consisted of giving an annual subsidy to a doctor already in the hire of a mining company in exchange for his medical services to the settlers.[23] On this question, Lessard answered Martel: ". . . I believe that we will be able to arrive at a definitive arrangement with the Ministry of Colonization when the legislative term is finished and the special credits are voted."[24] These credits worth $10,000,000 were finally voted in April 1935; the provincial government was thus committed, in virtue of the Vautrin Plan, to subsidize all aspects of the establishment and maintenance of settlers on the land,[25] calculating that, after a few years, these people would be able to support themselves. The Ministry of Colonization became then an autonomous ministry, and in October of the same year the decision as to medical services for settlers became the responsibility of this ministry rather than of the PBH. Indeed, in a circular addressed to the heads of health districts of the province, J. E. Caron, director of services, announced the fact that "Our department [Colonization] will pay from now on the bills of doctors who treat our needy settlers in settlements where there is no organized medical service."[26] This instruction, which conforms to the resolution reproduced in the Vautrin Plan, was, however, limited in nature; for example, a doctor's visit had first to be recommended by the head of the County Health Unit, who also had to initial all doctors' bills, which had to be finally approved by the PBH before the doctors could be paid. Also, these payments were only made for needy settlers. "We cannot of course extend such spending to farmers,"[27] Caron added. The projected plan, far from the solution that Martel had suggested they test at Duparquet, was almost impossible to apply in settlement areas given the vast distances involved, the urgency of some cases that required immediate attention, and the necessity of distinguishing between indigent settlers and often very poor farmers. Funds earmarked for medical aid to settlers being so limited, doctors continued to shun these regions.

Consequently, in December 1935 an alternative began to be seriously considered; the correspondence exchanged between the principal actors during that month gives a general idea of the pressures that were exerted. On 4 December 1935, Martel expressed in a letter to Lessard his desire to "discuss with the competent authorities this increasingly important question" of "the organization of Medical Service to Settlers," a subject for which, he assured, he possessed "a rather complete dossier."[28] The next day, Father Désilets, posted at Fréchette near Saint-Clément de Montbeillard in Abitibi, told the director of the PBH about a rumor to the effect that the government was going to set up one nurse in each parish.[29] In his first reply, Lessard toned down the priest's enthusiasm, but given the latter's insistence, he intimated in another letter a few days later that he was to see Martel shortly to discuss with him a plan for medical services in Abitibi.[30] From an exchange of five letters[31] between Lessard and Martel we know that the ball was in the court of the Ministry of Colonization and that a much awaited meeting was held in Québec on the 24 December 1935 at which the director of the PBH and the authorities of the Ministry of Colonization were present to discuss the project submitted by Martel, who also participated in the discussions. The plan proposed by Martel is unfortunately not in the archives; we do not know therefore to what extent it resembled the solution proposed for Duparquet. Events which follow show, however, that it was "the most reasonable solution" that carried the day on Christmas Eve 1935. We have not located the minutes of this meeting nor any official document that refers to it. We have also looked in vain for a law which instituted the MSS in a maze of legislative measures, and yet, the creation of each County Health Unit was instituted by orders in council. We are thus forced to try to reconstitute the most probable scenario that led to the establishment of the MSS and that explains its particular status and function in the social and health services structure of the period.

WHEN NECESSITY BECOMES THE LAWMAKER . . .

The meeting of 24 December 1935 was crucial because it brought together the representatives of government institutions that shared the responsibility of finding a solution to the lack of medical services in settlements (the Ministry of Colonization, the Provincial Bureau of Health, and the Bureau of Public Charities) and an individual who was capable of representing the daily reality of settlers: Martel. The problem that these people had to solve could very well appear unsolvable; yet, some compromise had to be found that could accommodate existing laws and respond to the needs created by the economic depression.

It is easy to imagine the arguments put forward in favor of "the most reasonable solution"; some of these had been stated by Lessard at the conference in 1934. One thing that had to be taken into consideration was that the normal application of the act regulating public charity did not permit payment of hospitalization fees for indigent people who lived in an unorganized territory. This act, passed in 1921, stipulated that hospitalization fees for indigent persons must be shared equally by the province, the municipality, and the hospital in question. However, as Lessard pointed out, the settlements were not organized municipalities and did not therefore have the power to collect the tax ("the poorman's penny") destined to finance a third of hospitalization fees. This state of affairs had caused problems for the provincial government during the initial settlements of the Gordon Plan, which had not made provisions for any medical service, and many settlers were sick and had to be hospitalized, the costs of which were assumed by the BPC.[32] Faced with this problem, the Ministry of Colonization at first agreed, following upon the suggestion of Lessard, that all aspiring settlers pass a medical exam before being selected for the settlements, an essential yet insufficient measure because:

> . . . female settlers, there as elsewhere, bear children and need services at times; there as elsewhere, there are accidents; there as elsewhere, there are epidemics or pulmonary disorders, diseases which require urgent care.[33]

However, nothing in the Québec Public Charities Act allowed for the dispensation of medical services, an argument against subsidies to doctors. Article 16 is particularly clear:

> The assistance accorded by government cannot, in any case, surpass one-third of the total cost of the maintenance of needy people taken in by a public charity institution.[34]

The act did, however, make provisions for certain measures for exceptional cases since, through article 17, it gave the government some leeway:

> The lieutenant governor in council may, nonetheless, upon recommendation from the bureau of public charities, in urgent and absolutely necessary cases, assist in a manner which he may judge appropriate the development of the work of public charity in the province.[35]

Thus there remained to be found the most "appropriate" manner to answer the urgent needs of the settlers in terms of health services. Here "the most reasonable solution" is all the more pertinent because the services of nurses, contrary to those provided by doctors, could be considered as minimal assistance to the needy. It is probable that the original idea to set up these nurses in residential dispensaries was but an extension of the concept of the dispensaries established in the cities of the 19th century in order to give specialized medical services to the poor.[36]

A fourth argument in favor of setting up nurses in residential dispensaries could be put forward. Indeed, the BPC had already supported dispensaries for the poor in the cities since it had recognized at its inception in 1921 certain specialized dispensaries as public charity institutions for special targeted clientele in large cities, mainly mothers and children. In these dispensaries, notably the antivenereal type, the service applied the principle of the Red Cross to the effect that ". . . dispensaries are open not only to the indigent poor but also generally to persons with but modest means."[37] One of the goals pursued was to reduce the hospitalization costs of the indigent poor whose state of health did not require hospitalization. However, how could one justify the generalization of such institutions to the settlement territories? We think that by committing himself to financing the nursing posts in the settlements, Lessard, in his capacity of director of the BPC, succeeded in persuading the representatives of the Ministry of Colonization to finance, at least until the creation of the Ministry of Health and Welfare,[38] the construction and maintenance of the residential dispensaries.

There remained the problem of how to supervise the nurses from an administrative and legal standpoint; one last argument could be brought forward. Certain measures contained in the act concerning the PBH and the act concerning County Health Units could be used. The 1922 act concerning the PBH had made provisions for appointing hygiene officers in unorganized territories, leaving to these officers the definition of their powers.[39] By virtue of this measure, Martel had been appointed medical officer in charge of the supervision of the settlement nurses in 1933. In the same year the act concerning County Health Units ensured the permanence of these organizations ". . . destined to supervise and protect public health in the counties where they are established."[40] The residential dispensaries in the settlements could thus be under the authority of the officer assigned to unorganized territories (Martel) or, by default, under the medical officer of the county's health unit. In either case, the MSS could be set up even though no law existed to that effect.

We think that it was essentially on the measures contained in the three above mentioned acts that the protagonists of the MSS relied in order to initiate and maintain the service. It appears evident that they did not want to invoke these measures to pay doctors, no doubt because the sums demanded by the latter were too high in the context of the Depression and because they knew doctors did not want to go into "exile" in the regions.[41] Unfortunately, the meeting of 24 December 1935 did not eliminate all the obstacles to "the most reasonable solution"; it merely authorized its discrete establishment. It would take several trials and errors before the MSS, essentially conceived as a nursing service despite its name, was officially created.

The Establishment of the MSS: From Improvisation to Official Recognition (1936–1943)

As early as January 1936, the authorities recognized that health services for settlers should be in the hands of nurses rather than doctors.[42] In February of the same year a rudimentary structure was set up through which the MSS could begin to function. However, it was not known how the system would work, that is, how the three institutions involved (the PBH, the BPC, and the Ministry of Colonization) would share financial and managerial responsibilities, a situation that led to a series of trials and errors. After 7 years of testing, the MSS became an official division of the Ministry of Health with its own regulations.

THE STRUCTURE OF "THE MOST REASONABLE SOLUTION"
In February 1936 "the most reasonable solution" became somewhat formalized since, on the 17 February, Martel sent a letter simultaneously to Lessard and to "all the Nurses and Doctors presently in Service in the Settlements" in which he first informed all interested parties of the status of the MSS "not yet definitely organized on a permanent basis." He explained that Lessard had put

him in charge "of setting up this new service," the functioning of which he briefly described through the use that the addressees must make of the forms MSS 1, 2, 3, 4, and 5. He ended his letter by asking them ". . . and to relieve the congestion of the Service at Québec, please send all correspondence that you used to send to this address, to my office at Amos."[43]

Beginning in February 1936 then the nurses received a copy of the forms for use in the service (MSS 1, 2, 3, 4, and 5) of which the first three "will take effect immediately." An examination of form MSS 1 shows that it was but a means of applying article 17 of the Public Charities Act; that is, it was an attestation that a person, deemed indigent, should be hospitalized at the expense of the BPC. Figure 1 allows for a better understanding of the particular status and functions of the Medical Service to Settlers.

From Figure 1 it is clear that the hospitalization fees of settlers were accepted by the BPC using public charity funds; it should be specified here that in order to apply the act concerning the Québec Bureau of Public Charities, the provincial secretary acted as minister. This simple form not only allowed settlement nurses to hospitalize a settler but it also allowed this to be done at the expense of the State! The MSS 2 form was used upon leaving the hospital.

Provincial Secretariat
Bureau of Public Charities
Government Place
Québec

Township, Settlement no. _____

Date:

To the Direction of _____ Hospital

Please accept for treatment at the expense of the Public Charity [P] who suffers from (probable diagnostic)

signed: _____
        (doctor or nurse)

A copy of this request for hospitalization must be transmitted simultaneously to the Bureau of Public Charities at Québec and to Dr. Martel in Amos.

Figure 1. Medical service to settlers form 1.

The MSS 3 form was quite different; it consisted of a one-page list of nurses' activities under twelve large headings: (1) maternal hygiene, (2) infant hygiene, (3) school hygiene, (4) contagious diseases, (5) tuberculosis, (6) vaccinations/ immunizations, (7) general medicine, (8) minor surgery, (9) dental care, (10) obstetrics, (11) doctors' visits, and (12) hospitalization. This form was used by nurses for several years to produce the weekly reports that they sent to Martel in Amos and Lessard in Québec. It is clear that all these operations performed by the nurses and reported under these headings surpassed the limits of "absolute necessity." As for forms MSS 4 and MSS 5, Dr. Martel only mentioned that "They are doctors' reports"; we only found one copy in the archives.

On 12 November 1936 the act that created the Ministry of Health and Social Welfare included in the same administrative structure the PBH (health) and the BPC (welfare) by permitting office holders "To favor, by all measures and means which they judge adequate, the advancement and development of public health in the province."[44] Furthermore, this act made it their "duty" to prolong life and avoid death. Up to the creation of this ministry, settlement nurses were hired by Lessard in his capacity as director of the Bureau of Public Charities, then, from the fall of 1936, by Nadeau, acting director of the Ministry of Health, and then by Dr. Jean Gregoire, Deputy Minister of Health from 1937 to 1962. In the organization chart of the Ministry of Health of 1938, the MSS was under the authority of the deputy minister and was placed under the heading "Medical Aid," which was subdivided into two parts "Indigent Poor of the North Shore" and "Settlers."[45] This rudimentary structure together with the temporary character of the MSS, created to respond to urgent needs, often forced the authorities to improvise.

AN UNDERSTANDABLE IMPROVISATION

The administrative improvisation that characterized the MSS during its first years of existence was often exasperating for nurses. It may be explained, however, by a relative negligence of the Ministry of Colonization and by the constant necessity of demonstrating the needs in order to obtain adequate budgets.

It seems clear enough that 1936 was a year of negotiations between the institutions involved. The BPC tried to avoid responsibility for the construction and maintenance of the dispensaries and for transportation and other material concerns while it took care of the nurses' salaries as well as the allocations to doctors who assisted the nurses when needed. On the 13 January

1936, in a typical letter of engagement addressed to Jeanne Chabot, Lessard explained the ambiguous situation at the start of the year:

> . . . it has now been decided that you will be with the Bureau of Public Charities from 15 December 1935 at a salary of $100.00 per month. It is to be understood that this is a temporary position which will last as long as we must maintain free Medical Service to Settlers and as long as your services are found to be satisfactory. As soon as we have finished our negotiations with the Ministry of Colonization, I will write again to you to explain your terms of engagement and give you the necessary instructions. You will then be under the immediate supervision of Dr. Émile Martel, medical officer at our Health Unit in the county of Abitibi who will be responsible for Medical Service to Settlers in Abitibi-Témiscamingue. . . .[46]

The letter of engagement of Marguerite Turgeon, dated 18 September 1936, seems to indicate that the negotiations were finished because it is more explicit than earlier letters concerning the shared responsibilities between the BPC and the Ministry of Colonization:

> . . . Your salary will be $100.00 per month beginning on the 21st September 1936 but you must look after your own board. Matters of housing, furniture, maintenance, heating, lighting and transportation will be taken care of by the Ministry of Colonization.[47]

During the first years the construction and maintenance of the dispensaries were constant worries. For example, in the letter of engagement of the nurse at Bellecombe, we read: "I think that before long, the Ministry of Colonization will give the necessary instructions for the construction and furnishings of the residential dispensaries for our nurses."[48] Yet, Bégin, the nurse posted at Rollet (Rivière Solitaire) since 1932, still lived in October 1936 in a "cabin" that "does not deserve to be called a dispensary"; she had to get her water "by the pail at the river!"[49] It was not only in matters of housing that the Ministry of Colonization neglected its responsibilities. Thus nurse Marguerite Patry wrote to Lessard, 8 May 1936, her fourth letter since the beginning of the year, in which she asked for a horse:

> . . . I have walked a lot along poor roads, in mud up to my knees. It looks like no decision has been made on the question of a horse for this summer. And yet, the department of colonization could very well spend something on this, it has done so on so many other rather more useless things than this.[50]

In May 1936 the MSS was located in the office of the Amos County Health Unit, but its budget was separate from that of the latter.[51] The letterhead carried the title "Provincial Secretariat—Public Charities Division—Medical Service to Settlers" because most of the funds that supported the MSS came directly from the Provincial Secretariat. Since it was a service for the indigent poor which relied essentially on the act concerning the Québec Bureau of Public Charities, its director had, at least once a year, to demonstrate its urgency and necessity in order to obtain the money necessary for its maintenance and expansion. This obligation led to numerous letters and papers, especially from the deputy minister Grégoire, which ensured special budgets were voted coming from the consolidated funds of the province. For example, on two occasions in 1941, Grégoire had to ask the Treasury Department for advances from the budget to pay unexpected expenses; two orders in council were adopted by the legislature, first on 16 July[52] and then on 9 October. The order in council of 16 July also stated that the budget voted on for the purpose of operating nurses' dispensaries had already been taken out of the Public Charities fund for several years past.[53] It thus allowed for the maintenance of twenty-four dispensaries in Abitibi, thirteen in Témiscamingue, six in the Saguenay, and ten others spread across Québec. Again in 1943, Grégoire invoked urgency and necessity when he pleaded to his superior that the Treasury Department not reduce from $74,000 to $55,000 the grant needed for:

> . . . the construction, maintenance and fitting out of our nurses' dispensaries in the settlements and in isolated regions. . . . These are cases of real necessity. . . .[54]

This requirement of constantly demonstrating the urgency and necessity of needs introduced a system of management that consisted of reacting to pressure from the settlements rather than one of planning for these needs. However, the authorities introduced gradually rules and regulations that became more and more formalized as the MSS expanded.

FROM TRIAL AND ERROR TO REGULATIONS

With the creation of the Ministry of Health the hiring and working conditions of the settlement nurses became somewhat standardized, first in a typical letter of engagement of six items that stood for a contract and then in the regulations, of which the first edition goes back to April 1942 and the last to February 1956. However, despite these efforts to standardize procedures and nurses' working conditions, the nurses often suffered the consequences of unpredictable problems.

Typically, the letter of engagement began with a paragraph informing the nurse of her appointment "by the Honorable Minister of Health and Social

Welfare to do public health work and provide health care to indigent settlers" while indicating the date at which she was to begin as well as the name of the settlement assigned to her.[55] The first item of the "contract" indicates the monthly salary; the nurse is also informed of the responsibilities of the Ministry of Colonization as stated earlier. After that the contract stipulates that the nurse will have surgical instruments "as well as a certain number of the usual drugs" with the warning "that no extravagant use is to be made of the drugs." At item three, the nurse learned that she should "ask for a reasonable amount for the drugs"; the sums thus collected had to be handed over to Martel.[56] Paragraph 4 of the letter described the necessary precautions in order to avoid abuses by the population:

> In order to avoid abuses, you must inform the population you are serving, by the priest or otherwise, that you are at their service for consultations at the dispensary in the morning for all patients who are not bedridden and who are, therefore, capable of coming to you. For patients who you must visit at their homes in the afternoon, let it be known that night calls must be avoided when there is no absolute emergency and let it be known by all the means at your disposal that we may remove their nurse at any time if we judge that there are uncontrollable abuses.[57]

Item five of the letter instructed nurses to send a weekly report of their activities to Martel. The sixth and last item consisted of a formal recommendation to "try to keep the hospitalization of patients to a strict minimum." It is particularly interesting because, in order to be able to better judge the urgency and necessity of hospitalization, the authorities came to explicitly request from the nurses a medical diagnosis! This instruction became an article in the Regulations for Medical Service to Settlers still in force in 1956: "Nurses . . . must not fill in the request for hospitalization form unless they have first . . . made a summary diagnosis."[58]

The nurses would discover at their own expense that these rules were easier to formulate than to apply. The correspondence exchanged between the nurses and the authorities during these years demonstrates the numerous problems that they had: unhealthy housing, supply problems of many kinds, notably of firewood and drinking water, problems in getting expenses reimbursed for the transportation of patients or for drugs administered, etc. We have already pointed out that the Ministry of Colonization did not always live up to its responsibilities; consequently, the nurses tended to take their problems to the Ministry of Health. This ministry ended up taking charge of nurses' housing and other expenses in 1939. However, the nurses were not always treated better by the Ministry of Health than by the Ministry of Colonization. For example, in 1938 the former refused to reimburse the travel expenses incurred by Marie-Louise Gagnon, nurse at Beaucanton, for an exceptional case. She had had to travel three times to assist in childbirth; the mother suffered from a psychological disorder, and the husband was epileptic. These very poor people had next to nothing; they used potato sacks for bed covers. The nurse had to pay for her meals, which she took at a neighbor's, and for her transportation, expenses of more than $8.[59] Despite the support of Martel the deputy minister responded that the Bureau of Public Charities could not foot the bill.[60] With time the nurses learned to get the transportation of patients authorized beforehand. Thus the nurses at Sainte-Thérèse-du-Colombier, a village between Forestville and Baie-Comeau, had often to request by telegram the authorization to transport by plane or by boat patients who needed to be hospitalized.[61]

The behavior of the authorities with respect to the cost of drugs was as ambiguous as their instructions. Indeed, while pharmaceutical and other medical products were furnished sparingly at the beginning, they were, theoretically, charged to users at the end of 1936 or at the start of 1937. In practice, many nurses accumulated unpaid bills for drugs that they had to buy themselves and get delivered by the large pharmacies of the urban centers. This situation became particularly frustrating in 1939 when the nurses' monthly salary was cut by 20%, bad news which prompted Lemieux to complain "that the settlers are often incapable of paying for the remedies, medical care and transportation. The product of my work is insufficient to cover these expenses. . . ."[61]

In 1943 the MSS became a division of the Ministry of Health and moved to Québec. The director, Martel, produced his first annual report, which, in its French version, only took up three pages of the report of the ministry. This first account of activities only concerned the dispensaries in Abitibi-Témiscamingue; it is therein stated that "The year 1943 was one of general organization for the Medical Service to Settlers" and that there were thirty-nine posts of the MSS in Abitibi and in Témiscamingue of which "the occupants were 38 nurses and one doctor."[63]

Conclusion

Necessity is the mother of invention; this saying is confirmed in the case of the creation of the Medical Service to Settlers. Constantly hearing the needs of the colonizing priests and of the settlers themselves, limited by legislation that reserved exclusively for doctors certain operations that they could not perform because they were absent, and limited by the budgets of the Great Depression, the authorities involved did, nonetheless, find a compromise solution acceptable to all parties concerned.

Using the leeway that certain existing laws provided and taking their inspiration from the dispensaries introduced in the cities in the 19th century, the protagonists of the MSS concocted a solution that was deemed reasonable and satisfactory by a sufficient number of people such that it was maintained well after the depression. The success of this solution came from the settlement nurses, the main actors in the system. Their competence, their generosity, and their devotion allowed for minimal assistance services to be offered to the indigent poor at an acceptable cost; by their ability to plead the urgency and necessity for intervention they ensured that thousands of poor people living far form urban centers could benefit from health services that otherwise would not have been accessible.[64]

In Canada and specifically, Québec, several commissions of inquiry have studied the question of accessibility to health services in remote regions from the point of view of the unequal distribution of doctors in the field.[65] Doctors' disdain for rural areas, not to mention remote regions, constitutes a problem that, although admitted by all and well documented, has yet to be satisfactorily solved despite certain efforts made in this sense since the 1930s.[66] The solution chosen by the government of Québec in the 1930s shows similarities with solutions adopted by at least three other provinces (Alberta, Saskatchewan, and Newfoundland), also confronted by the problem of accessibility to doctors in certain regions. The numerous studies in progress on nursing services in Canada and elsewhere in the world will eventually allow us to pinpoint the specificity of the case of Québec and permit comparisons.[67]

NICOLE ROUSSEAU, PhD
Professor
Faculté de Sciences Infirmières
Université Laval
Sainte-Foy
Québec, Canada G1K 7P4

JOHANNE DAIGLE, PhD
Associate Professor
Départment d'histoire
Université Laval
Sainte-Foy
Québec, Canada G1K 7P4

Acknowledgments

This research has been made possible by two grants from the Human Sciences Research Council of Canada (882-92-0029 and 816-95-0020). We wish to thank Francine Saillant, Ph.D. (Departement d'anthropologie, U. Laval) for the original idea for this project and for her participation in its initial stages. Our thanks also to Ghislaine Hebert, research professional, Guylaine Girouard, and David Pankow, research assistants, Departement d'histoire and Dominique Boudreau and Manon Henri, research assistants, Faculte des sciences infirmieres, U. Laval. Finally, special thanks to two partners associated with this project: The Order of Nurses of Québec and the Corporation du dispensaire de la garde, La Come, Abitibi. Translated from the original French by Robert Grace.

Notes

1. According to the dictionary, the word dispensary denotes "A charitable institution, where medicines are dispensed and medical advice given gratis, or for a small charge." *The Oxford English Dictionary*, 2nd ed., s.v. "dispensary." A dispensary is therefore a place where medical services are given. However, in the context of this article, the word refers both to the workplace and residence of the nurses; hence the phrase "residential dispensary," preferred by the successive authors of the annual reports of the MSS However, in a study on Social Security submitted to the Royal Commission of Inquiry on Constitutional Problems in 1955, Francois-Albert Angers claimed: "Each of these posts is a dispensary." Francois-Albert Angers, "La sécurité sociale et les problemes constitutionnels," app. 3, in the Report of the *Royal Commission of Inquiry on Constitutional Problems (Tremblay Commission)*, vol. II (Québec, 1955), 112.

2. Such was the case for Aylmer Sound, on the north shore, opened in 1986.

3. Here are a few more distances that will help to explain the isolation of the colonies: Montréal-Matane (northeast), 636 km; Montréal-Sept-Iles (North shore), 904 km; Val-d'Or-Rouyn-Noranda (west), 109 km; and Val-d'Or-Chibougamau (north), 396 km. It is also important to mention that, in the 1930s, proper roads were virtually nonexistent; many colonies could only be accessed by trails or by the railway.

4. There exist a few anecdotal pieces that show the role played by the settlement nurses. Among these the most important were those of Aurore Bégin published in the *Bulletin des Gardes-Malades Catholiques* between 1934 and 1941 and of Louis-Émile Hudon in the *Bulletin des Infirmieres Catholiques du Canada*, 12, no. 6 (1945): 182–190. Robert Germain devotes a few lines to the subject in "Le mouvement infirmier au Québec," in *Cinquante ans d'Histoire* (Montréal: Bellarmin, 1985), 31–32. A few missionaries and nurses relate in storybook form their experiences in the settlements of certain regions of Québec. See, in particular, Louis Garnier, *Du cométique à l'Avion: Les Pères Eudistes sur la Côte Nord (1903–1946)* (Québec: A. D'Amours, 1947); and Bérith Nicole (Dionne de la Chevrotière), *Rocabérant ou les Tribulations d'Une Jeune*

Infirmière Chez les Pionniers de l'Abitibi (Montréal: Éditions Sondec, 1974); also Marie Lefranc, *La Rivière Solitaire* (Paris: Ferenczi, 1934).

5. Garnier, *Les Pères Eudistes*, Dr. Alphonse Lessard (director of the Provincial Bureau of Health [PBH]; to Hector Laferté (Minister of Colonization), 29 December, box 4 File 1, Affaires Sociales: Dispensaires, Service Medical aux Colons, Archives Nationales du Québec (hereafter cited as SMC, ANQ, see note 6.

6. This article is based essentially on the following sources: (1) SMC, ANQ; it contains 9 boxes, each with several dossiers. We shall refer to these by the letters B and D to indicate the box and dossier in question. (2) Affaires Sociales: Unités sanitaires, Unité sanitaire Abitibi, Archives Nationales du Québec (hereafter cited as US, ANQ). (3) An unclassified collection available at the Région de l'Abitibi-Témiscamingue, Archives Nationales du Québec (hereafter cited as AT, ANQ). (4) The annual reports of the Medical Service to Settlers (MSS), published from 1943 to 1971 by the provincial Ministry of Health. We also did 48 interviews with as many nurses, either retired or still on the job, on the north shore and in Abitibi, as well as 24 interviews with people living in Abitibi-Témiscamingue who had recourse to the services of the settlement nurses; these interviews have not, however, been included in the preparation of this article.

7. There appears to have been one in Lamorandière in 1917 and another in Desmeloïze in 1921, two areas opened to colonization in the Abitibi region.

8. Garnier, *Les Pères Eudistes*, 185.

9. Georges Desrosiers, *Benoît Gaumer et Othmar Keel, La Santé publique au Québec: Histoire des Unités Sanitaires de comté 1926–1975* (Montréal: Les Presses de l'Université de Montréal, 1998). The PBH was under the jurisdiction of the Provincial Secretary.

10. Medical Inspection Report Dr. L. P. Savoie to Lessard, 5 September 1924, box 1, File 3, SMC, ANQ. Dr. Savote was responsible for this medical inspection. After having spent two months on the north shore over the summer of 1924 he concluded that, generally speaking, the people he met with had no notion whatsoever of basic hygiene.

11. Garnier, *Les Pères Eudistes*, 193.

12. Lessard to Lafertè, 29 December 1932, box 4, File 1, SMC, ANQ.

13. Raoul Blanchard, *L'Ouest du Canada Français* (Montréal: Beauchemin, 1954); Roger Barette "Le plan Vautrin et l'Abitibi-Témiscamingue," in *L'Abbittibbi et le Témiscaming*, ed. Maurice Asselin and Benoît Beaudry-Gourd (Hier et aujourd'hui, Rouyn, vol. 2: Département d'histoire et de géographic, 1975), 105–110; Michel Pelletier and Yves Vaillancourt, *Les Politiques Sociales et les Travailleurs*, vol. II, *Les Années 1930* (Montréal: published by the author, 1975), 247–66; Esdras Minville, "La législation ouvrière et le régime social dans la province de Québec," app. 5, in *Commission Royale des Relations Entre le Dominion et les Provinces*, (Ottawa: The King's Printer, 1939), 98.

14. Lessard to Laferté, box 4, File 1, SMC, ANQ.

15. Dr. Émile Nadeau, deputy director of the PBH, to Nurse Blais of Auclair, 14 January 1933, box 4, File 1, SMC, ANQ.

16. Michel Pelletier and Yves Vaillancourt, *Les Politiques Sociales et les Travailleurs*, vol. I, *Les Années 1900–1929* (Montréal: published by the author, 1974), 98. It should be noted that the Bureau of Public Charities constantly ran a deficit in the 1930s as

recalled by Gonzalve Poulin, "L'Évolution de l' assistance au Québec, 1608–1951," app. A in *The Report of the Royal Commission of Inquiry on Constitutional Problems (Tremblay Commisssion)* (Québec, 1955), 204. See also the study by Serge Mongeau, *Évolution de l'assistance au Québec* (Montréal: Le Jour, 1967), 123.

17. Several authors note the debate on this question such as Blanchard, *L'Ouest du Canada;* Barette, *L'Abbittibbi*; and Pelletier and Vaillancourt, *Les Politiques.* The Honorable Irenée Vautrin (Minister of Colonization), *The Acts of the Conference of Colonization Held at Québec, 17 and 18 October 1934* (Québec, 1935), gives a general idea of the several facets of the project submitted by the new Minister of Colonization.

18. *Le Devoir*, 9 August 1934.

19. Aware of the powerful influence of the clergy in Québec at that time, the government had specially convened the bishops and the colonization missionaries to this conference. Representatives of the settlement medical societies, but, to our knowledge, not of the nurses' association were also present.

20. Vautrin, Acts of the Conference on Colonization, 215–16.

21. Ibid., 216.

22. Ibid., 241–42.

23. Dr. Émile Martel to Lessard, 18 February 1935, box 1, File 1, US, ANQ.

24. Lessard to Martel, Québec, 23 February 1935, box 1, File 1, US, ANQ.

25. Pelletier and Vaillancourt, *Les Politiques,* 253–55.

26. J. E. Caron (director of services, Ministry of Colonization) circular to heads of [Health] Districts, 28 October 1935, box 1, File 1, US, ANQ. Following this instruction, Lessard specifies to Martel that "this question of medical service in the new settlements is the responsibility of the Ministry of Colonization and we are only acting as advisors. Consequently, you may advise interested parties to contact direct the Ministry of Colonization and we will cooperate if so desired." Lessard to Martel, Québec, 29 October 1935, box 1, File 1, US, ANQ.

27. Caron, box 1, File 1, US, ANQ.

28. Martel to Lessard, 4 December 1935, box 1, File 1, US, ANQ.

29. Father Désilets to Lessard, Saint-Clément de Montbeillard, 5 December 1935, box 4, File 4, SMC, ANQ.

30. Lessard to Désilets, Québec, 19 December 1935, box 4, File 4, SMC, ANQ.

31. Lessard to Martel, medical officer, Health Unit for Abitibi county, 11 December 1935, box 1, File 1, US, ANQ; Martel to Lessard, 13 December 1935, box 1, File 1, US, ANQ; Lessard to Martel, 17 December 1935, box 1, file 1, US, ANQ; Lessard to Martel, 18 December 1935, box 1, File 1, US, ANQ. There are two letters from Lessard to Martel dated 18 December; in one of these letters, Lessard invites Martel to come to Québec on 24 December to discuss the project. In the other letter he writes "Since the Ministry of Colonization decides, we could search for complementary information from its representatives. I am thinking of Ivanhoe Caron, colonizing priest and organizer, amongst others, in the service of assistance to settlers in this ministry between 1911 and 1923."

32. Vautrin, Acts of the Conference on Colonization, 215.

33. Ibid., 214.

34. "An Act respecting the Québec Bureau of Public Charities," in *Revised Statutes of the Province of Québec,* vol. III, chap. 189, art. 14–16 (Québec, 1925).

35. Ibid., art. 17.

36. Denis Goulet and André Paradis, *Trois siècles d'histoire médicale au Québec: Chronologie des institutions et des pratiques (1639–1939)* (Montréal: VLB Éditeur, 1992).

37. A.H. Deloges (director), and J.A. Ranger (assistant director), Venereal Disease Division, *Report of the Secretary and Registrar of the Province of Québec for the Year 1921–1922* (Québec: The King's Printer, 1922), 106.

38. It should be noted that the MSS set up 9 months before the creation of the Ministry of Health.

39. "An Act respecting the Québec Bureau of Public Charities," in *Revised Statutes of the Province of Québec, 1941*, chap. 138, art. 138 (Québec: The King's Printer, 1941).

40. "Act respecting County Health Units," in *Revised Statutes of the Province of Québec, 1941*, chap. 184, art. 3 (Québec: The King's Printer, 1941).

41. Two other authors have a similar interpretation of the known facts: Claire Martin, "L'Infirmière de colonie en Abitibi-Témiscamingue," historical narrative presented by the Corporation "Le dispensaire de la garde", La Come, Abitibi, to the Ministry of Cultural Affairs, Abitibi-Témiscamingue Directorate, Programme of Assistance to Organizations in Matters of Heritage, fall 1992; Angers, Royal Commission, vol. II, app. 3 (1955).

42. The hope of recruiting doctors remained, nevertheless, tenacious for awhile but, by February 1937, in his response to Father André Dumas, who had for a long time been asking for the services of a doctor for his parishioners, Émile Nadeau admitted: "You know that the honorable Minister of Health made an urgent appeal to doctors that they might offer their services. I must tell you that these offers are rather few in number and even rarer are those offers coming from doctors who are competent, sober, honest and conscientious." Émile Nadeau (acting director of the Ministry of Health), to Brother André Dumas (parish priest of Beaudry), 1 February 1937, box 4, File 4, SMC, ANQ.

43. Martel to Lessard, 17 February 1936, "Circular Letter," box 2, File 2, SMC, ANQ; Martel to Miss Jeanne Chabot (Nurse at Sainte-Gertrude, Abitibi), 17 February 1936, AT, ANQ.

44. "An Act respecting the department of health and social welfare," in *Revised Statutes of the Province of Québec, 1941*, chap. 182, sec. I, art. 3 (Québec: 1941). For convenience and because the documents consulted always refer to it in these terms from 1936, we shall use the term, "Ministry of Health."

45. Minville, "Le législation."

46. Lessard (director of the BPC) to Chabot (Sainte-Gertrude, Québec), 13 January 1936, AT, ANQ. It should be noted that this nurse had already been working in this settlement since at least 18 December 1935, the date of her first weekly report sent to her superior.

47. Lessard (director of the BPC) to Marguerite Turgeon, September 1936, AT, ANQ. It should be specified here that, in principle, the settlers themselves were to supply the nurse with firewood.

48. Lessard (director of the PBH) to Marguerite Patry, 23 January 1936, box 2, File 2, SMC, ANQ.

49. Ministry of Health, n.d., box 4, File 5, SMC, ANQ; Martel, "Report on the dispensary at Rollet," 14 October 1936, box 4, File 5, SMC, ANQ.

50. Patry to Lessard (Bellecombe), 8 May 1936, box 2, File 2, SMC, ANQ. While it is unclear whether the Ministry of Colonization was supposed to assume costs related to transportation, it is clear that the Ministry of Health never wanted this responsibility. Dr. Jean Grégoire (Deputy Minister of Health) to Father Dubois (parish priest of Saint-Roch-Bellecombe), 24 January 1939, box 2, File 2, SMC, ANQ. An examination of the reports of the Ministry of Colonization has shown that they are more or less silent on the Medical Service to Settlers and the settlement nurses. In defense of the Ministry it ought to be noted that its total annual subsidy went from $5,657,340. in 1939 to $671,479 in 1944.

51. Up until then the correspondence of the Medical Service to Settlers carried either the letterhead of the Bureau of Public Charities (BPC) or that of the PBH, as revealed by the study by Martin, "L'Infirmière de colonie," p. 13. With respect to the budget, Martel received the following instruction from the director of the PBH on 3 April 1936: "As concerns your expenses for settlers' medical care, charge them to a different account [from that of the Health Unit] and we have asked the Treasury Department for an advance of $150.00 from the Public Charities fund . . . ," Lessard to Martel, 3 April 1936, box 1, File 1, US, ANQ.

52. Order in Council, Executive Council Chambers 1809, Québec, 16 July 1941.

53. Ibid., second para.

54. Grégoire, "Paper for the Honorable Mr. Henri Groulx," 21 October 1943, box 1, File 1, SMC, ANQ.

55. See among others the letters of engagement of Marguerite Turgeon, 18 September 1936; Marcelle Gingras, 30 December 1936; Jeannette Beaumier, 26 May 1937; and Irène Adam, 7 December 1942, available at the AT, ANQ.

56. Nadeau (acting director, Ministry of Health) to Marcelle Gingras (nurse in the township of Castagnier, Québec), 30 December 1936, AT, ANQ.

57. Grégoire to Irene Adam (nurse at St-Nazaire de Berry, Québec), 7 December 1942, AT, ANQ.

58. Armand Laberge (temporary Assistant Deputy Minister, acting director, Medical Service to Settlers) *Rules and Regulations for Employees of the Medical Service to Settlers,* art. 61 (Québec: Ministry of Health of the Province of Québec, 1 February 1956), p. 9.

59. Marie-Louise Gagnon to Martel, 11 September 1938, box 4, File 9, SMC, ANQ.

60. Grégoire to Martel, 3 October, 1938, box 4, File 9, SMC, ANQ.

61. Telegram from Louise Matte (nurse at Ste-Thérèse-du-Colombier) to Grégoire, 12 February 1941 at 4:45 P.M., box 3, File 1, SMC, ANQ; Telegram from Matte to Grégoire, 22 September 1941 at 8:05 P.M., box 3, File 1, SMC, ANQ.

62. Murielle Lemieux to Grégoire, Rollet, 20 March 1939, box 4, File 5, SMC, ANQ.

63. Martel, Director, Division of the Medical Service to Settlers, "First Annual Report," in *Second Report of the Ministry of Health for the Years 1941, 1942 and 1943* (Québec: Ministry of Health and Social Welfare, 1995), 306.

64. It is worth mentioning that, as a mark of appreciation of the settlement nurses work, the La Corne dispensary in Abitibi was recognized as an historic site and officially opened on 24 June 1997; it had been occupied by nurse Gertrude Duchemin from 1936 to 1976.

65. *Report of Inquiry on Health Services (Sylvestre Report)* (Québec: 1948); *Report of the Royal Commission of Inquiry on Health and Social Services (Rochon Commission)* (Québec: 1987).

66. Some of the various solutions proposed include a guaranteed minimum revenue for doctors practicing in isolated communities, the establishment of mobile medical units, and the relaxation of laws that prevent foreign doctors from practicing outside of university hospitals. This last solution even became an issue in the 1994 election in Québec when a group of "doctors without borders for isolated regions" held a hunger strike in order to obtain government authorization to practice their profession in remote regions.

67. For Alberta, see Sharon Richardson, "Political women, professional nurses and the creation of Alberta's District Nursing Service, 1919–1925," *Nursing History Review,* 6 (1998): 25–50; Sharon Richardson, "Frontier Health Care: Alberta's District Nursing Service, 1919–1976" (paper presented at the annual conference of the Canadian Society for the History of Medicine, Memorial University, St. John's, Newfoundland, 8 June 1997). For Ontario, see C. Commachio-Abeele "'The Mothers of the Land Must Suffer': Child and Maternal Welfare in Rural and Outpost Ontario," *Ontario History* 80 (1988): 184; C. Commachio-Abeele, "'Nations Are Built of Babies', Saving Ontario's Mothers and Children, 1900–1940," (Montréal and Kingston: McGill-Queen's University Press, 1993), 340; Meryn Stuart, "Ideology and Experience: Public Health Nursing and the Ontario Rural Child Welfare Project, 1920–1925," *Canadian Bulletin of Medical History/Bulletin Canadien d'Histoire de la Médecine* 6 (1989): 111–131. Nancy Edgecombe from Yellowknife, "The Evolution of Nursing in the Northwest Territories" (paper presented at the Canadian Association for the History of Nursing, International History of Nursing Conference, Vancouver, 12–15 June 1997); and Jeanette A. Klotz from Rockhampton, "They Also Serve Who Stand and Wait-Remote Area Nurses at Birdsville, Australia, 1939–1945" (paper presented at the Canadian Association foe the History of Nursing, International History of Nursity Conference, Vancouver, 12–15 June 1997) show a growing interest for the study of nursing services in regions that lack doctors.

To Cultivate a Feeling of Confidence
The Nursing of Obstetric Patients, 1890–1940

SYLVIA RINKER

Department of Nursing
Lynchburg College

Mothers of infants born at the end of the 19th century in America were the first to receive the assistance of the "trained obstetrical nurse."[1] Throughout the first half of the 20th century the nurses who cared for obstetric patients were charged with managing patients, their families, and their surroundings to make possible the aseptic delivery required by a growing medical science. Caring for new mothers who gave birth at home and later in hospitals, the pragmatic nurses of the first half of the 20th century were actively involved in developing an obstetric nursing practice that espoused the traditional nursing values of caring and compassion but also bore clear marks of the growing medical and obstetric science of the time.[2] In 1915, nurse Sara Bower stated emphatically that it was a particular responsibility of the nurse to "cultivate at all times a feeling of confidence in the patient."[3] However, as historian Judith Leavitt argued, new mothers who were submitted to the rigid scientific care of the era reported feeling not confidence but rather a sense of being left "alone among strangers."[4] Leavitt has offered a thoughtful analysis of this discrepancy, but further exploration of the problem is needed.[5]

Historical investigation into the evolution of clinical practice offers insight into the conflict between science and nurturing that erupted as nursing ideals confronted the everyday experiences of the nurses and patients involved. Tensions between the nurse's role as a scientific manager and her expected function as a nurturing caregiver were evident at the outset of professional nursing; a century later the dialectic tension between the scientific base of nursing and its moral base of care remains unresolved.[6] Nurses shaped their practice by choosing actions from those that were possible within the context of the time.[7] The clinical practice nurses developed, viewed as an outcome of

Nursing History Review 8 (2000): 117–142. A publication of the American Association for the History of Nursing. Copyright © 2000 Springer Publishing Company.

choices made, provides evidence that offers insight into the continuing ambiguity of the historical role of nurses expected to function as both scientific and caring practitioners.[8]

"Filling the gap between home and hospital adequately," and "smoothing the path for the obstetric art" were duties that the nurse, as an early 19th-century woman, was peculiarly qualified to perform. Recruited because she was a woman, the newly emerging "trained nurse" was charged with the task of convincing women to abandon the familiar female-surrounded birth-at-home experience in favor of the rapidly growing scientific medical childbirth in the hospital.[9] Dr. Joseph B. DeLee, a dominant figure in American obstetrics at the turn of the 20th century, prescribed a specific role for the nurse explicitly designed to benefit the new obstetric "specialty" and its physician practitioners.[10] He said:

> The nurse may do much to aid the physician in obtaining from the public that recognition for obstetrics that the specialty so justly deserves. Thus, the nurse may smooth the path for the advance of the obstetric art. She becomes really a missionary spreading the gospel of good obstetrics.[11]

As defined by the influential DeLee, childbirth required that strict limits, imposed by scientific asepsis rules, be applied to nursing practice. Thus, from the outset the nurse's innate female attributes, governed by the scientific principles of obstetric medicine, constituted the foundations for both the power and the limits of obstetric nursing. Welcoming the status afforded by their association with the newly emerging specialist obstetricians, nurses readily accepted a role that they were only partially able to define. Charged with delivering scientific care, the nurse remained on the periphery in defining the dimensions of that care.[12]

Societal Forces

Obstetric nursing grew out of social forces in America in the early 20th century that combined to define birth as a medical event and propelled its move into the hospital. Industrialization and urbanization promoted the growth of institutions for birth. While the Progressive Era gave rise to the expectation that better health and living conditions for women and infants were both necessary and possible, confounding high maternal and infant mortalities continued to defy medical science throughout the period. Childbirth killed five times as many women aged 15–44 as did typhoid fever, and only tuberculosis outranked parturition as a killer of women in 1917.[13] Maternal mortality rates averaged over 60 per 10,000 throughout the period of this study and did not begin a steady downward trend until 1934, when sulfonamides became available to treat deadly puerperal infections.[14] During this time a prenatal emphasis developed also, in an attempt to curb infant mortality, thus expanding the physician's domain to include the scientific management of the woman before birth as well as at the delivery and beyond.[15] Attempts to cope with the desperate conditions of the Great Depression brought radical changes in government support for healthcare, and insurance became available to pay hospital costs. All of these factors combined to propel birth into the hospital, creating the need for skilled nurses to care for obstetric patients.[16]

The belief in the power of science held by Progressive Era Americans to improve the lives of citizens and the growing power of the medical profession made the association of nursing with medicine an attractive alliance to nurse leaders.[17] Eager to promote nursing as a respectable profession, Isabel Hampton referred to the nurse as the "physician's lieutenant," who, by virtue of her training, was "allotted a part to perform in the progress of medical science."[18] Hampton's vision of the possibilities for nursing included a clear commitment to standards, precision, and method for the organization, teaching, and practice of nursing.[19] Speaking at the Chicago World's Fair in 1893, and demonstrating her understanding that working within the system could strengthen the position of the nursing profession, Hampton willingly accepted a limited role for nurses, as she said: "To be sure, the nurse is only the handmaid of that great and beautiful medical science in whose temple she may only serve in minor parts."[20]

The rapid growth of hospitals and the system that developed for the employment of nurses fostered both the educational and economic dependence of nurses on physicians. Initially taught by physicians, student nurses at the turn of the century were indoctrinated into a hierarchy that made the nurse responsible not to the patient but to the physician. Because hospitals used pupil nurses to care for patients and did not employ graduate nurses until the 1930s, nurses had to rely primarily on the referrals from physicians for their private duty nursing cases after graduation. Novice nurses who, until the 1930s, were primarily students in the hospitals had neither the knowledge nor the authority to question a nursing practice that accepted a subordinate role dictated by medicine.[21] Anxious to establish themselves as valuable assistants to physicians, nurses developed a practice that gave priority to medical science and the needs of physicians over the needs of individual patients. Scientific principles provided the foundation for the beginning practice of obstetric nursing and directly affected the relationships nurses established with their patients. Georgina Pope, Superintendent of Nurses at the Columbia Hospital for Women in Washington, DC, underscored the central role of the nurse and her value as a scientific practitioner when she said, "It is through the nurse that the doctor expects to combat the frightful disease of puerperal fever . . . she can become of no less importance than the physician himself in guarding the health and preserving the lives of mothers and children."[22]

Certainly the life-threatening danger of puerperal sepsis colored the evolution of obstetric nursing. Oliver Wendell Holmes had published his classic article "On the Contagiousness of Puerperal Fever" in 1843, and by 1879, Louis Pasteur had demonstrated that the infectious streptococcus was responsible for puerperal fever.[23] Science had provided a way, through antiseptic and aseptic practices, to overcome the killer, and its principles must *not* be violated. In 1924, Dr. Charles Reed, speaking to the Illinois State Association of Graduate Nurses, identified the "foundational qualities" of the nurse to be courage, tenderness, and self-control. He continued:

> and yet, though she have the courage of a lioness, the divine tenderness of a mother, and the self-control of a Capulet, and have not science, it shall profit her nothing. Her training in science, science clear, precise, inevitable, is the necessary medium through which her mind and emotions express themselves. It is the master tool of her profession.[24]

The traditional nursing values of compassion, comfort, and support for the whole person clashed with the rigors of scientific asepsis that defined the medical practice of obstetrics; the nursing care that developed bore the marks of this conflict.

Obstetric Nursing in Home Deliveries

Despite an active campaign conducted by physicians to promote hospital birth in the early decades of the 20th century, in 1940, half of all deliveries in the United States still occurred at home.[25] Once the pregnancy was confirmed, the mother-to-be usually initiated an employment interview with the prospective nurse.[26] While it was common for the physician to recommend private duty nurses for employment, in obstetric cases the situation was often reversed. The nurse was key to promoting medical care for childbirth at the turn of the century because, just as women had felt comfortable in approaching the female midwife in the past, many women contacted the nurse before selecting their physicians.[27] Katharine DeWitt urged the private duty nurse whose patient had not yet consulted with a physician to offer to go with the patient to the doctor's office or come to the house when the doctor was first summoned if "nervousness" were the reason that the woman had postponed her initial contact with a physician. DeWitt loyally followed DeLee's dictates that when available, specialist obstetricians be employed as birth attendants because "a nurse can never forget what complications may arise requiring the greatest skill obtainable."[28]

The nurse who assisted at an operative delivery in the home faced a task of daunting proportions.[29] A nurse's tactful ability to secure the patient's cooperation was as crucial as her scientific training because she was required to convert the patient's private home into an aseptic field for scientific birth.[30] Building a trusting relationship with her patient was an essential first step as the nurse was responsible for convincing the mother that it was necessary to scrub all floors, walls, and furniture and otherwise rearrange the family's furnishings for birth. She must ensure that all equipment was sterile and at hand. After the environment was cleansed the nurse was expected to wash thoroughly her patient also, both internally and externally.[31] A warm bath, soapsuds enema, and in the early years an antiseptic douche were followed by additional scrubbing of the skin from the breasts to the knees, including the perineum, the buttocks, and the thighs.[32] Perineal shaving, begun in the early decades of the 20th century, continued, despite its demonstrated futility, well into the 1980s.[33] Following the cleansing, the mother-to-be was placed in an elaborately prepared bed for her labor. The nurse's responsibility then was to remain with her patient and send for the doctor when delivery was imminent.[34]

Considerable skill was required to comfort and reassure women who were normally frightened and anxious at the onset of labor. Graduate nurses who were experienced in the care of childbearing women recognized the value of the personal relationship with their patients. Nurse Louella Adkins wrote in 1903: "A thorough acquaintance of the peculiarities of each patient is a wonderful help, and should be sought in all ways short of inquisitiveness before the confinement."[35] She believed that the "well-bred observance of the patient is the guide to the *unobtrusive control* which the successful nurse must exercise."[36] The nurse who functioned autonomously to help her patient accept medical interventions for birth and maintain self-control throughout the ordeal of labor not only facilitated aseptic deliveries, she also made the entire experience much more pleasant for the physician and the family.

As nurses soon learned, developing good relationships with physicians was also essential for a pleasant birthing experience. According to Nurse Mary Keith the "wise" nurse had consulted with the physician before labor to find out when he wished to be notified.[37] Central to ensuring a safe delivery, the nurse must use her scientific knowledge to judge when to send for the physician. At the same time that such clinical judgments were expected of the nurse, she was cautioned repeatedly not to diagnose because diagnosing was considered exclusive medical territory.[38] The nurse was to inform the physician of the condition of his patient,

> without giving her opinions. It is the duty of the nurse to inform the doctor that there is some antepartum flowing, for instance, or that the uterine tumor bulges sideways . . . but it is not her business to suspect aloud that it is a case of placenta previa, or a transverse position of the child.[39]

The nurse's tact and flexibility were essential to provide safe care to the patient while maintaining the appropriate medical hierarchy. A certain amount of finesse was also required for the procedure of notifying the physician to come for the delivery: "The nurse should know enough never to send peremptorily for the doctor when there is no immediate necessity."[40]

A very common occurrence in home births was the arrival of the infant before the physician. Distances between patients' homes, difficulty in delivering messages, and their other patient responsibilities all prevented the physician's presence at the moment of birth. This was especially true in rural areas. Studies by the Children's Bureau reported repeatedly that even in the rare event when a physician had been engaged to attend births, he usually did not arrive in time.[41] The competent, adaptable nurse functioned in the doctor's presence as his "assistant"; in his absence, she functioned as the previously noted "lieutenant."[42] In recognition of this fact, nursing textbooks of the period gave instructions to the nurse first on her delivery duties in the physician's absence and then on her tasks in his presence.

Inherent in the nurse's role was preventing the unwarranted disturbance of the physician. The doctor's role was to manage the birth, not the labor leading up to the birth.[43] Dr. Stanley Warren saw "no intrinsic fitness in the obstetrician serving as a watchful nurse at the bedside forty-eight hours before he is wanted."[44] Clara Weeks-Shaw, author of an early nursing textbook, gave fair warning: "Perhaps more often in obstetric cases than in any others, the nurse is called upon to assume, in his absence, responsibilities properly belonging to the physician."[45] Some private duty nurses refused to take obstetric patients for this very reason.[46] Although uncomfortable with the responsibility for managing birth, the nurses who took obstetric cases did accept the delivery as part of their role as valuable helpers to the physician.[47] According to A. Worcester the "best assistants are those who themselves are able to take charge."[48] By limiting the types of cases she took, a nurse developed her expertise and could claim to be a "specialist" in obstetric nursing just as the physician had become a specialist by limiting his practice to obstetrics. A major reason obstetric nurses were embraced by scientific medicine while lay mid-wives were not is that nurses were always careful to recognize and protect the physician's authority even when fulfilling duties that were properly defined as medical obligations. The obstetric nurse accepted a dependent role, sanctioned by the authority of scientific medicine, that midwives refused. By assuming the delivery duty without the decision-making power to determine how the birth should be managed, nurses became firmly entrenched as subordinates in the medical sphere.[49] By accepting responsibility for managing the delivery, defined by medical science as strictly within the medical domain, nurses made themselves central to a process they had little authority to define or control.

Nurses quickly became indispensable assistants in providing the scientific medical advantage of anesthesia to women at birth.[50] Hampton encouraged nurses to use every opportunity while in training in the hospital to prepare themselves for giving anesthetics when they became private duty nurses in homes.[51] DeLee wrote in 1907 that since the doctor frequently prescribed chloroform the nurse should know the procedure well because "when the child is coming through the vulva, the nurse may have to administer the chloro-form."[52] The nurse's duties while giving anesthesia included protecting the patient's face from the irritating vapors by smearing vaseline around the patient's mouth and nostrils, dripping the anesthetic on a handkerchief or an ether cone held over her face, and watching the patient's pulse and facial appearance very carefully for untoward signs.[53] The nurse was to give her full attention to this responsibility as the life of mother and infant were literally in her hands.[54]

Following delivery of the infant and the placenta, the responsibility for preserving the newly delivered mother's life landed squarely on the nurse's shoulders. In the first hours after delivery the nurse's "vigilant watchfulness offered the only security."[55] The nurse's observation of signs and symptoms were pivotal for safe medical care, and there was no question that the nurse was held responsible for the accurate interpretation of signs and the ultimate fate of her patient. In 1916, Nurse A. Young literally saved her newly delivered patient's life by her alert assessment of the deteriorating vital signs that followed the high forceps delivery of her patient.[56] Left alone to monitor her patient's recovery following delivery, she called the physician back to the home when it became clear to her that the patient must be transferred to the hospital for a life-saving blood transfusion and surgical repair of a hemorrhaging cervical tear. Young continued to care for the patient, carefully recording her vital signs, during the course of her hospitalization. At the end of 3 weeks, Young reported that "in spite of all Mrs. A. had gone through, there was no infection, and mother and baby left the hospital in good condition." Young demonstrated a sophisticated understanding of the pathophysiology involved in the medical treatment of postpartum hemorrhage. Scientific medical care, though admittedly the probable cause of the cervical tear that led to the hemorrhage in the first place, eventually saved this mother's life. Because of the nurse's intelligent, rapid response to her patient's deteriorating condition, the medical care she desperately needed had the opportunity to be successful.

The medical treatment receives center stage in Young's account of her experience, while the nursing care that made it possible is not recorded. Any emotional support and care given as nurse and family faced the trauma of an emergency transfer from the home to the hospital and the potentially imminent death of the mother were not part of the record she published in the professional journal. Instead, the authoritative knowledge of scientific medicine was the knowledge this nurse deemed important to document. The clinical judgments nurses made on the basis of their scientific observations clearly differentiated professional nurses from untrained attendants. In the developing profession of nursing, documenting the contributions of nurses to medical practice was a first step necessary for the acknowledgment of nurses as skilled professionals. In the evolution of nursing, expertise in the application of scientific medical knowledge was foundational for the future acceptance of the profession as a legitimate partner with medicine.

Nurses learned their lessons well; gaining scientific knowledge and experience, they began to evaluate the performance of physicians. When necessary, well-trained scientific nurses took the responsibility to ensure safe medical practice. Bower described a home delivery in 1915 at which it was her "painful duty and professional privilege" to protect her patient from a lax physician.[57] She reported that when he arrived, the physician had, "incredible as it may seem, fingernails that were black, absolutely filthy." By providing scrub brushes, pouring water, placing solutions where he could hardly avoid them, and using "mental suggestion" with all her force, Bower successfully protected her patient against infection. Proud of her practice, she said: "I came out victorious, a clean baby, and a complete and happy recovery." In 1915, with a maternal mortality rate of over 60 per 10,000 and an infant mortality rate of over 100 per 1,000, a safe recovery from childbirth was no mean accomplishment.

In addition to interpreting strictly scientific principles, graduate nurses proved to be very capable of actively translating their scientific knowledge into actions that could be safely adapted to the individual situations of their patients. Adkins was convinced, in 1903, that "Good antiseptic technique could be carried out in a barnyard, if the brain that directs it is trained in principles and details."[58] On the subject of care of the newborn's cord she said:

> If we know we want to desiccate the cord as quickly as possible, and remember that any liquid put upon it will delay that result, we will be rewarded by a clean little pink dimple, whether we keep the stump clean and dry with the daintiest absorbent cotton, or with the scorched, and therefor sterile rag of the old-time nurse.

The nurse's ability to individualize the scientific care prescribed by medicine was important to the development of nursing as a profession with its own approach to patient care.

The patient record of a mother who did not survive her birth experience offers an example of nursing practice that combined the best available scientific medical care with the nurturing new mothers expected from their nurses. Susan Moore's pregnancy ended abruptly on June 4, 1908, when she suddenly began having the first of a series of convulsions that eventually required her admission to Columbia Hospital for Women in Washington, DC.[59] The best medical care and medications were unable to stop the convulsions, and Moore's infant was delivered, via high forceps, stillborn.[60] Within the nurse's postpartum notes are many medical assessments, including frequent recordings of the patient's temperature that spiked to 105° 5 days after delivery. Repeated doses of strychnine, laxatives, and whiskey were given, along with oxygen, in desperate attempts to save the patient's life. Nurses' observations, "respirations very rapid and painful; complaining of pain in left side; sighing a good deal in sleep; quite restless, seems very uncomfortable; very bad wheezing in chest; talked irrationally greater part of night; seems brighter this morning" documented in the nurses' notes, indicate the close attention her nurses paid to caring for this mother.[61] On the night before Moore died the nurse on duty wrote: "Does not want to be alone." One of the last nursing actions recorded, in the face of imminent death, was the placement of a hot water bottle on to the patient's left side. Nearly comatose, she could not have directed this action. No doubt the nurse had remembered Moore's earlier complaints of pain in her left side.

Within an hour the patient's respirations had ceased. The scientific observations documented by Moore's nurses were important for helping physicians decide on the medical treatment she would receive. The nurses' recordings of Moore's responses to various medicines and treatments give evidence that nurses' actions were based not only on physicians' orders, but also on their own interpretations of the comforting measures Moore needed.

Obstetric Nursing in Hospital Births

The gradual movement of birth from the home to the hospital gained momentum as the 20th century progressed. Mothers who delivered in hospitals before 1920 were primarily single or indigent women; however, by the mid-1920s, Americans had begun to see hospitalized birth, as well as hospitalization for other conditions, as symbolic of economic and social status.[62] Nationwide the 37% of hospital births that occurred in 1936 had grown to 55% in 1940 and by 1951 had reached 90%.[63] By the 1930s a growing number of middle-class women, whose healthcare expenses were occasionally subsidized by insurance, began to choose hospitals for birth.[64] The hospital nursing staff also changed; beginning in the 1930s, student nurses were replaced by graduates employed as staff nurses.[65]

The hospitalization of birth facilitated a greater number and frequency of procedures that greatly increased nurses' duties. From 1890 to 1940 a dramatic increase in the "operative interventions" used for childbirth in hospitals is clearly evident. The use of forceps, induction via inflatable balloons, versions, episiotomies, and cesarean sections had all been available since the mid-19th century but were not widely used until the 20th century.[66] The overall operative intervention rate for deliveries at Columbia Hospital in Washington, DC, more than tripled from 20% in 1892 to 66% in 1920.[67] Sixty-five percent of the women who delivered at the Chicago Lying-In Hospital between 1918 and 1925 had operative deliveries; by 1931, 80% of women received some type of intervention for birth.[68]

The strict asepsis that nurses and physicians tried to uphold in home births was even more rigorously pursued in hospitals. Rigid routines were developed to streamline the extra care required by the growing population of patients who were receiving increasing numbers of interventions for their births. Physicians lent their authority, and nurses used it willingly to promote scientific birth restrictions. Asepsis rules required banning family and friends from the laboring rooms in the hospitals.[69] Dr. Anna Fullerton noted that the nurse "succeeds best" in this process by telling the friends that it is the doctor's wish that she exclude them.[70] Nurses willingly supported policies that separated a woman from her family on her admission to the hospital, stripped her of her clothes, shaved and purged her, and sometimes restrained her, all in the pursuit of asepsis.[71] Individualized care suffered under this regime and certainly contributed to the dissatisfaction among mothers that Leavitt documented.[72] The nurses who participated in such actions believed the scientific training they had received; they were convinced that such policies were justified to save mothers and infants from death. One 1937 graduate nurse reported: "Infection didn't stand a chance. We used Lysol solutions for perineal care and sprayed merthiolate on the perineum every time we could!"[73]

Second only to the fear of death in childbirth among women at the end of the 19th century was a nearly universal dread of pain.[74] American women actively sought anesthesia, offered as one of the chief advantages of scientific birth.[75] Mary Blackwell, R.N., understood the challenge and the prestige of nursing the medicated woman in labor when she observed in 1931, "the nursing care of obstetric patients having analgesia and anesthesia is a difficult, though interesting duty."[76] The nurse administered the medication and applied the restraints, changing in the process, as historian Margrete Sandelowski has noted, "from a sisterly companion to an unfeeling robot."[77] Birth became an event not to be accepted and celebrated but to be managed and controlled. Because the anesthetized, restless patient could give no warning of an impending birth, making precipitous delivery very likely, the nurse who managed such a process successfully was obviously an accomplished partner in scientific birth.

As at-home births, the good nurse in the hospital saved the physician's time by calling him at just the right moment for the delivery. She became skillful at preserving the peace by giving careful attention to maintaining the established hierarchy. One nurse who began her practice in the 1930s reported that she was always careful, in reporting her laboring patient's condition, not to make a medical diagnosis.[78] "I'd call the intern and tell him 'I think' the patient is ready for delivery," she said. The intern came, examined the patient, and "informed" the nurse of the patient's progress. The intern notified the resident, who appeared on the labor unit in time to tell the nurse to call the attending physician; then he gave the order to move the patient "immediately" to the delivery room. Within the hospital system the nurse's knowledge was validated only when confirmed by the physician's authority. Experienced nurses knew, however, how to manage the system so that inexperienced interns and residents made the right decisions. While the intern and resident were busy confirming what this nurse already knew, she had already notified the anesthetist, the scrub nurse, and the circulating nurse so that all could be "in the delivery room, lined up and ready to go" before the attending physician arrived. That she managed, repeatedly, to get all of the personnel in their proper places at the right time, without ruffling feathers, was an accomplishment that this nurse reported with obvious pride, 50 years after the fact! Central to the action that facilitated a smooth delivery, the nurse kept her "place" by allowing the interns and residents to pronounce the medical judgments she had already made and acted upon. The mother was safely delivered, and the nurse's position as a valuable assistant within the system was maintained.

By giving priority to science and the physician over individual attention to the patient the nurse compromised the traditional woman-to-woman connection that had made her so valuable a missionary of the gospel of good obstetrics. Once the public had been convinced to accept medical attendance at birth, the womanly attributes of the nurse were redirected to support physicians and medical procedures rather than the patient who was giving birth. As good missionaries, obstetric nurses believed the gospel that strict adherence to asepsis principles was requisite to saving the lives of mothers and babies. As there could be no tolerance for breaks in aseptic technique, there could be no deviation in the hospital routine that might permit the introduction of the infectious germ. The hard-fought battle against maternal mortality was just beginning to lower the death rates of mothers in the late 1930s, and despite patients' complaints, nurses were convinced that the rigid policies were justified to protect their patients.

Conflict: Managing the System and Sustaining the Patient

Charged with spreading the gospel of good obstetrics, nurses discovered that their management skills were necessary to keep the household functioning during the disruption caused by scientific birth. As domestic managers in the hospitals, nurses were also responsible for promoting the smooth, efficient running of the institution. Nurses became adept at the scientific management of equipment, patients, and personnel in the hospitals. The priority for nursing care remained, throughout the time period of this study, to "smooth the path" for the physician and to ensure the economic efficiency of the hospital.

As hospitals changed from charity institutions to business enterprises, efficiency was prized for its economic value as well as for its influence on the happiness of physicians.[79] Beginning in the 1920s, caught in an ever greater push for hospital efficiency and economy, nurses participated in time-motion studies of nursing procedures and divided nursing care into component parts.[80] In the process the sympathetic, womanly qualities, so crucial for the acceptance of medical birth, were submerged under a scientific mold that required conformity and a standardized approach to patient care. Nurses developed and published clearly delineated standards and procedures in professional journals that reflected the values of the developing profession. The "Stewart Standards," used for evaluating nursing techniques in the 1930s included safety for patient and nurse; therapeutic effect; comfort and happiness of the patient; economy of energy, time, and materials; adaptability of the procedure to new situations; and the artistic, finished appearance of the work.[81] Detailed drawings in texts and journals showed *the* correct way to bind the abdomen and breasts following birth and *the* correct way to place instruments on a perineal care tray, and outlined strict schedules for maternal and infant elimination and feeding.[82] As they developed nursing procedures, questions about the relative merits of various solutions used for perineal care, about the most efficient breast care, and about what was the quickest way, compatible with safety and comfort, of getting twenty bedpans to twenty patients were all of concern to the developing professional nurses in the 1930s.[83] Articles published in journals of the time show that nurses were beginning to follow the medical model of scientific research to validate nursing interventions. Documenting the contributions of nurses to medical practice was a first step, necessary for the acknowledgment of nurses as skilled professionals. In the evolution of nursing, expertise in the application of scientific medical knowledge was foundational for the future recognition of nursing as a legitimate profession.

Permeating the asepsis and efficiency emphases, however, is evidence that nurses valued comforting, compassionate nursing actions that paid attention to their patients' human needs. Their scientific training provided nurses the building blocks for their practice, but as Carolyn Van Blarcom, one of the first nurses to write an obstetric nursing text in the 1920s noted, "No matter how well-trained or how complete the routines may be, the quality of the nurse's mind and the spirit that pervades her work are the determining factors in the effectiveness or futility of her endeavor."[84] The stereotypical approach required by medical asepsis created discomfort for mothers and conflict for nurses who were taught: "Sustaining the patient is the heart of the matter so far as nursing is concerned: the individual patient is the point. We see the problem from the patient's point of view so far as is humanly possible."[85] In the midst of burgeoning science and expanding technology, nurses recognized that comforting the patient was an appropriate, even expected, realm for nursing. The nurse's expertise in developing relationships with female patients was an important reason physicians enlisted nurses to promote medical care for childbirth in the first place. Speaking at the 1893 Chicago World's Congress, Pope said: "The mind of the pregnant woman is very susceptible to disturbing impressions, and the influence of a good nurse at such a time is immeasurable."[86] Although scientific efficiency and technical procedures clearly impinged on those relationships, nurses continued to recognize their interactions with patients as important for the delivery of effective nursing care. Practicing nurses clearly recognized that attention to patients' needs for emotional support was a crucial component of effective nursing practice. One wrote, "the nurse has not done well if she neglects to pay particular attention to the mental condition of the patient."[87]

Sustaining the patient required responding to patients' expressed needs. As time passed, new mothers became more vocal, clearly shaping the nursing care they received. Obstetric patients eventually changed the practice of the time that restricted newly delivered mothers to bedrest during the 10–14 days after their deliveries.[88] Initially, nurses tried to make new mothers follow the rules. However, nurses who were constantly with their patients during this long bedrest noted that the longer the patients stayed in bed, "the weaker they got."[89] One nurse noted that despite nurses' attempts to enforce doctors' orders, "you couldn't *keep* mothers in bed when they wanted to get up."[90] She reported that nurses just pretended not to see when patients got out of bed earlier than they were supposed to. Although physicians gave the orders, nurses decided when and where to enforce them, and the patients ultimately obeyed or not. Despite their position as dispensers of powerful medical science, doctors did not have total control. While physicians dictated what was to be done, nurses and patients began to define the manner in which medical treatments were accomplished, signaling an emerging sphere of nursing practice that emanated from a response to patient needs.

Nurse's Point of View

As nurses became more proficient in managing the details of aseptic delivery, they also promoted education that focused more specifically on nursing responsibilities. Physicians had been the first teachers in nursing schools, but by 1928, Jane McLaughlin wrote that nursing students needed instructors who could teach obstetrics "from the nurse's point of view."[91] This "nurse's point of view" included proficiency in medical assessments as well as a cognitive identification of the "art of nursing" or the manner in which skills were performed. Van Blarcom was particularly sensitive to the effect of the nurse as an empathetic supporter to the woman in labor: "this kind of assistance is indeed a comfort to the patient who appears to derive from it both a moral and physical sense of being helped in her struggle."[92] Not all nurses adopted the nurturing approach promoted by the leaders of the profession, but nurses were encouraged to "adopt a warm and sympathetic attitude" toward their patients.[93] Practicing obstetric nurses recognized that their ability to affect the mother's experience fell within the nurse's sphere of action. One nurse wrote, "I have found that if the mother is relaxed, contented, and happy, the baby will be a sleepy, contented baby awakening only long enough to take nourishment. I bend all my efforts in this direction."[94] Another noted, "The details of care, of course, are specified by the physician, but the effectiveness of the planning is largely dependent on the nurse's intelligence, interest, and conscientiousness."[95]

By 1940, nurses who worked in specific labor and delivery, postpartum, and nursery units began to develop a clinical expertise and familiarity with the routine that freed them to pay attention to patients' needs for comfort beyond the strict scientific application of medical treatments. In the process of smoothing the path for the advance of obstetrics, nurses had begun to develop a vision no longer confined to the field of medicine. While cooperative with medicine, nursing was moving beyond a physician definition of the function of nurses. Nurses lent their energy, intelligence, and abilities to promoting medical care for childbirth, but because of their relationships with patients, nurses were privileged to a particular kind of knowledge that while derived from and complementary to medical knowledge, was different. As the profession developed, nurses used their insights to shape nursing practice; the missionary began to craft her own message. Van Blarcom clearly stated: "Asepsis must come first and foremost, but the nurse's attitude and care of her patient must be mellowed by an always deepening sympathy and understanding." She continued:

> Good nursing implies more than the giving of bed baths and medicines, boiling instruments and serving meals. It is more than going on duty at a certain time, carrying out orders for a certain number of hours and going off duty again. It implies care and consideration of the patient as a human being and a determination to nurse her well and happily, no matter what this demands.[96]

While clearly acknowledging the physician as the authority, trained nurses began to identify specific areas that were the nurse's responsibility. In the process they also established nursing as a reputable profession with a sphere of practice that was complementary to, but separate from, that of physicians. In a subtle shift from the silent subservience of early practice, nurses began to participate in patient care discussions with physicians, in some instances presenting case studies at regularly scheduled conferences with physicians.[97] Using their knowledge and experience to discuss patient care, nurses began, formally, to define and develop nursing procedures. Navigating the shifting boundaries of science and nurture and struggling to meet the diverse expectations of patients, physicians, and hospital administrators, practicing nurses between 1890 and 1940 established the clinical practice of obstetric nursing as an integral component of medical care for birth.

Conclusion

The obstetric nurses of the first half of the 20th century fulfilled their mission to convince women of the need for medical attendance at birth. From a historical perspective the rigid scientific nursing of obstetric patients that developed by 1940 was a logical consequence of the circumstances within which it developed. The efficiency and efficacy that were the primary goals of obstetric nursing care in the 1920s and 1930s clearly conflicted with delivery of the individualized nursing care mothers needed and eventually demanded. Initially sought for their domestic abilities, nurses soon learned that scientific expertise gave them welcomed authority and prestige in the medical environment where they practiced.[98] Scientific expertise was the focus for the newly emerging profession of nursing, while the "deep sympathy of a woman" was an expected attribute, seen as a naturally occurring, particularly desirable characteristic of an obstetric nurse.[99] Nurses of the era would not have conceived there to be an incompatibility between science and nurturing. One was learned, and the other was expected. Both were requisite for the practice of professional nursing, but the history of clinical practice indicates that the prestigious scientific approach did take priority in the early years of nursing.

Convincing women to accept scientific birth and transforming homes and hospitals into aseptic environments required expert managerial abilities. The "tactful" nurse who could manage growing numbers of patients and physicians as well as the equipment for birth was valued as an accomplished professional. Nurses' skillful movement between their essential and ancillary positions smoothed the path for obstetrics, but also contributed to their invisibility within the early healthcare system. As a result, the nurturing relationship requisite for effective nursing and satisfied patients was also hidden, over-looked, and devalued. Historian Thomas Olson has documented that the "handling, managing, and controlling" abilities of students were the attributes praised by nursing superintendents between 1915 and 1937, while the "lan-guage of caring" was absent.[100] Historical investigation of the clinical outcome as real nurses translated ideal practices into the confines of everyday nursing, however, indicates that a fundamental source of nurses' power, knowledge, and influence was found in the relationships they established with their patients. Nearly a century ago, Bower recognized the significance of nurse-patient relationships when she identified that the nurses' primary duty was "to cultivate at all times a feeling of confidence in the patient." Her insight remains relevant today.

Across the ages (and across cultures), new mothers and their families have consistently identified nursing support as a primary ingredient for their satisfaction with childbirth care.[101] The human person-to-person connection, so easily taken for granted, was at the core of effective nursing in the first half of this century. Today, as burgeoning technology continues to require ever more technically proficient scientific practitioners, the problem of humanizing scientific care surfaces again and again.[102] Historical investigation of clinical practice indicates that nurses who would provide effective nursing care must temper needed scientific interventions with a compassionate approach that also nurtures patients' individual, human needs. At the outset of the new millennium, patients continue to need competent nurses who know how to give the best of scientific care by developing relationships that recognize and support the individual needs of patients.

Historical studies of the evolution of clinical practice have just begun. Examining the everyday practices of nurses in contact with patients has the potential to illuminate both productive strategies and limiting compromises nurses have made as practice has evolved. Over time, nurses' knowledge and expertise remained perversely hidden in the rush to meet the rapidly changing needs of an ever-evolving healthcare system. Exploration of the historical record can correct this picture by making explicit the distinct impact of nursing. What better source for evidence-based practice than the insights available from studying the documented outcomes of historical clinical prac-tice? The history of developing nursing practice in all clinical areas offers a rich source of data that has barely been tapped. Such research holds the potential to offer a deeper understanding of the ongoing paradoxes of the nursing profession—enduring dilemmas such as the tensions between nurture and science—that continue to confound questions about the nurse's proper function and role.[103] How nursing ideals were transmitted into everyday practice and the results of nurses' alliances with patients, families, and physicians are other areas that need to be explored. Investigating of the history of clinical practice, where nurses meet patients, warrants serious efforts from historians who wish to explore the complex history of nursing.

SYLVIA RINKER, RN, PhD
Associate Professor of Nursing
Department of Nursing
Lynchburg College
3527 Round Hill Road
Lynchburg, Virginia 24503

Notes

1. Herbert Stowe, "The Specially Trained Obstetric Nurse—Her Advantages and Field," *American Journal of Nursing* 10 (1910): 550–54 (hereafter cited as *AJN*). Nurses were educated and practiced as generalists. The term "obstetric nurse" in this paper does not indicate exclusive obstetric practice; it merely designates the title given the nurse while she cared for obstetric patients.

2. Diane Hamilton, "Constructing the Mind of Nursing," *Nursing History Review* 2 (1994): 3–28.

3. Sara Bower, "The Obstetrical Nurse," *AJN* 15 (June 1915): 734–35.

4. Judith Leavitt, "'Alone Among Strangers': Birth Moves to the Hospital," in *Brought to Bed: Childbearing in America 1750–1950* (New York: Oxford University Press, 1986).

5. Judith Leavitt, "'Strange Young Women on Errands': Obstetric Nursing Between Two Worlds," *Nursing History Review* 6 (1998): 3–24.

6. Alison Kitson, "Does Nursing Have a Future?," *Image* 29 (1997): 111–15.

7. Catherine Scholten, "'On the Importance of the Obstetrick Art': Changing Customs of Childbirth in America 1760–1825," in *Women and Health in America*, ed. Judith Leavitt (Madison, Wisc.: University of Wisconsin Press, 1984), 146. Judith Leavitt, "'Science' Enters the Birthing Room: Obstetrics in America Since the Eighteenth Century," *The Journal of American History* 70 (September 1983): 281–304; Herbert Thoms, *Our Obstetric Heritage: The Story of Safe Childbirth* (Hamden, Conn.: Shoe String Press, 1960), 93. John Duffy, *The Healers: A History of American Medicine* (Urbana, Ill.: University of Illinois, 1979).

8. Charles Rosenberg, "Clio and Caring: An Agenda for American Historians and Nursing," *Nursing Research* 26 (January/February 1987): 67–68.

9. Richard Wertz and Dorothy Wertz, *Lying-In,* expanded ed. (New Haven, Conn.: Yale University Press, 1989); Judith Leavitt, *Brought to Bed: Childbearing in America 1750–1950* (New York: Oxford University Press, 1986); Nancy Dye, "Modern Obstetrics and Working-Class Women: The New York Midwifery Dispensary, 1890–1920," *Journal of Social History* 20 (1987): 549–64.

10. For the first half of the 20th century, there was little agreement on what constituted an obstetrical specialist. The American Board of Obstetrics and Gynecology with requirements for specialty approval was established in 1930. Charlotte Borst, "The Professionalization of Obstetrics," in *Women, Health, and Medicine in America,* ed. Rima Apple (New Brunswick, N.J.: Rutgers University Press, 1992), 197–216. Joseph B. DeLee was born in 1869 and died in 1942. He wrote nearly 100 articles, 18 editions of *Obstetrics for Nurses,* first published in 1904, and 13 editions of *The Principles and Practice of Obstetrics,* first published in 1913. He founded the Maxwell Street Dispensary and Chicago Lying-In Hospital in 1895. By the time of his death in 1942 he had a well-earned reputation as a "formidable force in American obstetrics"; Judith Leavitt, "Joseph B. DeLee and the Practice of Preventive Obstetrics," *American Journal of Public Health* 78 (October 1988): 1353–60.

11. Joseph B. DeLee, *Obstetrics for Nurses,* 2nd ed. Philadelphia: W. B. Saunders, 1907), 18; and "The Prophylactic Forceps Operation," *American Journal of Obstetrics and Gynecology* 1 (1920): 34–44.

12. DeLee, *Obstetrics for Nurses;* Stowe "The Specially Trained Obstetric Nurse," 550.

13. U.S. Children's Bureau, *Save the Youngest: Seven Charts on Maternal and Infant Mortality, With Explanatory Comment* (Washington, D.C.: Government Printing Office, 1923), 2. In the United States, reliable birth and death statistics were not systematically collected until the Birth Registration Area was created in 1915. The first Birth Registration Area included ten states and the District of Columbia; it gradually expanded until all of the states were included by 1933. Harold Speert, *Obstetrics and Gynecology in America: A History* (Chicago: American College of Obstetricians and Gynecologists, 1980), 146.

14. Nancy Dye, "The Medicalization of Birth," in *The American Way of Birth,* ed. Pamela Eakins (Philadelphia: Temple University Press, 1986), 42. Not only did maternal mortality rates not decline, they actually increased an average of 0.4% each year from the 61 per 10,000 live births recorded in 1915 to the 65 per 10,000 rate of 1927. Irvine Loudon, "Maternal Mortality: 1880–1950—Some Regional and International Comparisons," *The Society for the Social History of Medicine* 1 *(1988)*: 183–228. Information is found in Kitson, "Does Nursing Have a Future?," 188; Irvine Loudon, "Maternal and Infant Mortality 1900–1960," *The Society for the Social History of Medicine* 3 (1991): 39. Current maternal mortality rates in the United States are 5–6 per 100,000 White women and 18–22 per 100,000 Black women per The Center for Disease Control, 3 September 1998.

15. The infant mortality rate, at a staggering 100 deaths per 1,000 live births in 1915, began a slow but steady decline to the 47-per-1,000-rate of 1940, per the Federal Security Agency, National Office of Vital Statistics, Louise Zabriskie, "Table 3: Trend of Infant Mortality in the United States Expanding Birth- Registration Area by States,

1915–1948," in *Nurses' Handbook of Obstetrics*, 9th ed. (Philadelphia: J. B. Lippincott, 1952), bound between pages 608 and 609; Richard Meckel, *Save the Babies: American Public Health Reform and the Prevention of Infant Mortality, 1850–1929* (Baltimore: Johns Hopkins University Press, 1990); Elizabeth Enochs, "Maternal Mortality: The Situation in Fifteen States," *The Trained Nurse and Hospital Review* (September 1934): 211–215.

16. Beth Rodgers, "The Great Depression, 1929–1940: An Era of Reform," *Virginia Nurse* (Spring 1984): 12–13; Ronald Numbers, "The Third Party: Health Insurance in America," in *Sickness and Health in America*, eds. Judith Leavitt and Ronald Numbers (Madison: University of Wisconsin Press, 1978), 142; Editor, "Better Times Ahead," *Hospitals* 10 (February 1936): 55; Phoebe Pollitt and Camille Reese, "Nursing and the New Deal: We Met the Challenge," *Public Health Nursing* 14 (December 1997): 373–82.

17. Robert Wiebe, *The Search for Order: 1877–1920* (New York: Hill and Wang, 1967); Leavitt, "Science Enters the Birthing Room," 303.

18. Isabel Hampton, "Educational Standards for Nurses," in *Nursing of the Sick 1893: Papers and Discussions from the International Congress of Charities, Corrections, and Philanthropy, Chicago 1893* (New York: National League of Nursing Education, 1949), 2.

19. Ellen Baer, "Nursing's Divided House—An Historical View," *Nursing Research* 34 (January/February 1985): 32–38.

20. Hampton, "Educational Standards," 2.

21. Patricia Benner, *From Novice to Expert* (Menlo Park, Calif.: Addison-Wesley, 1984).

22. Georgina Pope, "Obstetric Nursing," in *Nursing of the Sick 1893*, 166.

23. Oliver Wendell Holmes, "On the Contagiousness of Puerperal Fever," *The New England Quarterly Journal of Medicine and Surgery* VI (1842–1843): 503–30; See Elaine Larson, "Innovations in Health Care: Antisepsis as a Case Study," *The American Journal of Public Health* 79 (January 1989): 92–99, for a complete discussion of the controversy over the contagiousness of puerperal fever in the mid-19th century; Dorothy Lansing, Robert Penman, and Dorland Davis, "Puerperal Fever and the Group B Beta Hemolytic Streptococcus," *Bulletin of the History of Medicine* 57 (Spring 1983): 70–80.

24. Charles Reed, "Teaching Obstetrics to Student Nurses," *AJN* 24 (December 1924): 1210–11. Quote is on p. 1211.

25. Neal Devitt, "The Transition from Home to Hospital Birth in the United States, 1930–1960," *Birth and the Family Journal* 4 (Summer 1977): 47–58.

26. Katharine DeWitt, *Private Duty Nursing*, 2nd ed. (Philadelphia: Lippincott, 1917), 143. An oral history of the maternity portion of a private duty nurse's practice between 1934 and 1944 also documents this practice: Marian MacKinnon, "What a Difference a Nurse Makes—Then and Now," *Western Journal of Nursing Research* 19 (December 1997): 795–801.

27. In 1902 an obstetrician in Maine noted that only half of the patients in his experience had selected a physician before the delivery, while all of the women had chosen their nurses. Stanley Warren, "Technique of Labor in Private Practice," *American Journal of Obstetrics and Diseases of Women and Children* XLV (January 1902): 26–39.

28. DeWitt, *Private Duty Nursing,* 144.

29. Trained as generalists, graduate nurses, like medical students, often graduated with little practical experience in caring for maternity patients. The Committee on the Grading of Nursing Schools found that 18% of the nurses who had graduated in 1928 had had either "no practical experience or inadequate experience" in maternity nursing. The difficulty of predicting the timing of birth made it very likely that the private duty nurse on an obstetric case would have to deliver the infant herself before the physician arrived. May Burgess, *Nurses, Patients, and Pocketbooks* (New York: Committee on the Grading of Nursing Schools, 1928), 453.

30. See Pope, "Obstetric Nursing;" Henry Fry, "Obstetrical Emergencies," *AJN* 1 (November 1900): 107–11; Mary Keith, "Preliminaries of Obstetric Nursing," *AJN* 1 (January 1901): 257–59; Louella Adkins, "The Care of an Obstetrical Patient," *AJN* 3 (June 1903): 709–11, Jennie Putnam, "An Obstetrical Case at Home," *AJN* 10 (April 1910): 469–71; Elizabeth Burttle, "Obstetrical Nursing," *AJN* 16 (October 1915): 195–97; Louise Zabriskie, "Maternity Nursing in Hospital and Home," *AJN* 29 (October 1929):1157–64; Florina Carbone, "Obstetrics in the Home," *Trained Nurse and Hospital Review,* 95 (September 1935): 228–31. See also Isabel Hampton, *Nursing: Its Principles and Practice* (Philadelphia: Saunders,1893); Clara Weeks-Shaw, *Textbook of Nursing,* 3rd ed. (New York: D. Appleton & Co., 1912).

31. Pope, "Obstetric Nursing," 587; Keith, "Preliminaries of Obstetric Nursing," 258; Putnam, "Case at Home," 469; Hampton, *Nursing,* 368; and Weeks-Shaw, *Textbook of Nursing,* 275.

32. At the Cook County hospital in 1906 the vaginal douche was used before delivery. Henry Lewis, "Obstetrical Technique in the Cook County Hospital," *Surgery, Gynecology, and Obstetrics* 2 (January/June 1906): 81–82. See Pope, "Obstetric Nursing," 542; Anna Fullerton, *Handbook of Obstetric Nursing* 3rd ed. rev. (Philadelphia: P. Blakeston, Son, & Co., 1893), 70; Weeks-Shaw, *Textbook of Nursing,* 275.

33. R. Johnston and R. Siddall, "Is the Usual Method of Preparing Patients for Delivery Beneficial or Necessary?" *American Journal of Obstetrics and Gynecology* 4 (December 1922): 509–12; Mallie Montgomery, "An Obstetrial Case Study," *Trained Nurse and Hospital Review* 91 (September 1933): 245–51; Catherine Betz, "A Study of an Obstetrical Patient," *AJN* 34 (November 1934): 1109–16; Margaret Martin, "A Normal Mother and Baby," *AJN* 39 (October 1939): 1144–49; Karen Landry and Darla Kilpatrick, "Why Shave a Mother Before She Gives Birth?" *Maternal Child Nursing* 2 (May/June 1977): 189–190.

34. A. Worcester, "Obstetrical Nursing," *Boston Medical and Surgical Journal* CL (1904): 1–5; Pope, "Obstetric Nursing"; Fry, "Obstetrical Emergencies."

35. Adkins, "The Care of an Obstetrical Patient," 711.

36. Ibid.

37. Keith, "Preliminaries of Obstetric Nursing," 258.

38. Anne B., R.N. (1931 graduate of Youngstown Hospital School of Nursing), interview with author, Lynchburg, Va., 25 July 1994.

39. A. Worcester, *Monthly Nursing,* 2nd ed. (New York: Appleton, 1890*),* 46. The placenta previa is an implantation of the placenta low in the uterus that may cause bleeding or "antepartum flowing" in labor. A transverse position of the child in labor occurs when the presenting part is an arm or a shoulder.

40. Worcester, *Monthly Nursing,* 46.

41. See Frances Bradley and Margretta Williamson, *Rural Children in Selected Counties of North Carolina*, Publication No. 33 (Washington, D.C.: Government Printing Office, 1918); Elizabeth Moore, *Maternity and Infant Care in a Rural County in Kansas*, Publication No. 26 (Washington, D.C.: Government Printing Office, 1917); Florence Serbon and Elizabeth Moore, *Maternity and Infant Care in Two Rural Counties in Wisconsin*, Publication No. 46 (Washington, D.C.: Government Printing Office, 1919); Viola Paradise, *Maternity Care and the Welfare of Young Children in a Homesteading County in Montana*, Publication No. 34 (Washington, D.C., Government Printing Office, 1919).

42. A. Worcester, "District-Visiting Nursing in Obstetric Practice," *Boston Medical and Surgical Journal* 89 (December 1898): 539.

43. Fry, "Obstetrical Emergencies," 109.

44. Stanley Warren, "Technique of Labor in Private Practice," *American Journal of Obstetrics and Diseases of Women and Children* XLV (January 1902): 26–39. Quote is on p. 30.

45. Weeks-Shaw, *Textbook of Nursing*, 268.

46. Ninety-four percent of four thousand physicians in 1928 reported that they often needed a nurse for their obstetric cases. May Burgess, *Nurses, Patients, and Pocketbooks* (New York: Committee on the Grading of Nursing Schools, 1928). Of fifty graduate nurses surveyed in Kentucky in 1923, only 12% accepted obstetric cases. William McConnell, "The Trained Nurse in Obstetrics," *Southern Medical Journal* 16 (October 1923): 792–99. Other reasons given for refusing obstetric cases were that the work was too hard for the amount of money, too much time was lost waiting for women to be delivered, and some nurses "simply did not like this class of work."

47. One elderly nurse reported that she took a private duty case in a rural community, and while she knew what to do for a delivery, she reported that she was "praying hard" for the doctor to arrive before the baby. "He showed up," she said, "just as the head was born." Of course, the nurse had already made all the preparations needed, and while the delivery was completed smoothly and quickly, it was not without distress and anxiety for the nurse. Immediately following this experience, the nurse refused two other obstetrical cases even though she knew that to do so might place her on a "black list" and compromise her future earnings. R. Bland (R.N., 1937 graduate of Virginia Baptist Hospital), interview with author, Lynchburg, Va., 20 March 1994.

48. Worcester, *Monthly Nursing*, 65. Nurse authors Elizabeth Fishback, "Obstetrical Nursing as a Specialty," *AJN* 14 (July 1914): 806–11; Bower, "Obstetrical Nurse"; Burttle, "Obstetrical Nursing"; Keith, "Preliminaries of Obstetric Nursing," 257; Pope, "Obstetric Nursing"; and Adkins, "The Care of an Obstetrical Patient"; all addressed "obstetric nursing" as a specialty.

49. Margrete Sandelowski, *Pain, Pleasure, and American Childbirth* (Westport, Conn.: Greenwood Press, 1984), 70.

50. Fanny Longfellow delivered her third child with the benefit of ether in 1847 and thus became the first American woman to enjoy an anesthetized birth. She called ether "the greatest blessing of this age." Cynthia Pitcock and Richard Clark, "From Fanny to Fernand: The Development of Consumerism in Pain Control During the Birth Process," *American Journal of Obstetrics and Gynecology* 167 (September 1992): 581–87. Catholic sisters were the first nurses in America to administer anesthesia for

surgical operations, beginning in 1877. Marianne Bankert, *Watchful Care: A History of America's Nurse Anesthetists* (New York: Continuum, 1989), 25. John Duffy, "Anglo-American Reaction to Obstetrical Anesthesia," *Bulletin of the History of Medicine* 38 (January/February 1964): 32–44; Leavitt, *Brought to Bed;* and Sandelowski, *Pain, Pleasure, and American Childbirth* document the process of women demanding pain relief for childbirth in the early decades of the 20th century.

51. Hampton, *Nursing,* 331.

52. DeLee, *Obstetrics for Nurses,* 119.

53. Untoward signs included "the breathing or the pulse may suddenly cease and the face take on a livid hue or become ghastly pale." Hampton, *Nursing: Its Principles and Practice,* 338.

54. Nurses were instructed in 1912 to "Devote your sole attention to the anesthesia. Do not try to do or see anything else at the same time." Weeks-Shaw, *Textbook of Nursing,* 251.

55. Worcester, *Monthly Nursing,* 92.

56. A. Young, "Transfusion of Blood in an Obstetrical Case," *AJN* 17 (November 1916): 128–29.

57. Bower, "The Obstetrical Nurse," 735.

58. Adkins, "The Care of an Obstetrical Patient," 710.

59. Birth Record 416, in *Patient Records, April-June 1908,* Administrator's Office, Columbia Hospital for Women and Medical Center, Washington, D.C.

60. Chloral hydrate, veratrum viride, a spinal and arterial depressant, and strychnine sulfate, a tonic, affecting especially the nervous system, were all tried in futile attempts to stop the convulsions. Weeks-Shaw provides a useful list of "Drugs in Common Use," in, *Textbook of Nursing,* 139–53.

61. Although the notes are not signed, the changing handwriting in the medical record indicates nurses' shifts that varied in length from 7.5-14 hours.

62. One woman, born in 1921 at the Columbia Hospital for Women in Washington, D.C., recalled her mother saying how pleased she and her father had been "to have a doctor who specialized in obstetrics as well as a hospital that led the field in obstetrics and gynecology." Mrs. H.L.R., personal letter to the author, 5 November, 1993. Sixty percent of births occurred in hospitals in Washington, D.C., 63% occurred in Chicago, 65% occurred in St. Paul, and 77% occurred in Minneapolis by the mid-1920s. Dorothy Mendenhall, *What is Happening to Mothers and Babies in the District of Columbia?* (Washington, D.C.: Government Printing Office, 1928), 24; Editor, "Maternity, Child-Welfare and Social Service (in Chicago)," *Transactions of the American Hospital Association* 31 (1929): 31; Robert Woodbury, *Maternal Mortality: The Risk of Death in Childbirth From all Diseases Caused by Pregnancy and Confinement,* Children's Bureau Publication No. 158 (Washington, D.C.: Government Printing Office, 1926), 87; Fred Adair, *Prevention of Neonatal Mortality From the Obstetrician's Point of View,*(Washington, D.C.: Government Printing Office, 1929), 2.

63. Devitt, "The Transition", 47–58.

64. See Molly Ladd-Taylor, "'Grannies' and 'Spinsters': Midwife Education Under the Sheppard-Towner Act," *Journal of Social History* 22 (Winter 1988): 255–75; Rosemary Stevens, *In Sickness and in Wealth: American Hospitals in the Twentieth Century* (New York: Basic Books, 1989).

65. Marilyn Flood, "The Troubling Expedient: General Staff Nursing in United States Hospitals in the 1930s," (Ph.D. diss., University of California, Berkeley, 1981).

66. Mechanical induction involved the use of inflatable balloons pushed through the cervix or other instruments to forcibly dilate the cervix. Janet Ashford, "A History of Accouchement Force," *Birth* 13 (December 1986): 241–49. Version was a method of turning the infant in the uterus for a more favorable presentation for birth. Stephen Thacker and David Banta, "Benefits and Risks of Episiotomy: An Interpretive Review of the English Language Literature, 1860–1980," *Obstetrical and Gynecological Survey* 38 (1983): 322–38; Jane Sewell, *Cesarean Section—A Brief History* (Washington, D.C.: American College of Obstetricians and Gynecologists, 1993); Speert, *Obstetrics and Gynecology.*

67. Columbia Hospital, *Annual Reports of the Columbia Hospital for Women:* (Washington, D.C.: Columbia Hospital for Women and Medical Center.

68. *Statistical Report of the Chicago Lying-In Hospital and Dispensary,* Lying-In Hospital Records Collection, University of Chicago Library, Chicago, Ill., 1918–1925, 1925–1927, 1928–1931.

69. Interviews by the author with six nurses who practiced in the 1930s and 1940s and six mothers whose deliveries occurred by the 1940s reveal a consistent pattern in hospital births. All of the nurses interviewed stated that they were glad they had retired before husbands, families, and, as one declared, "anybody in the neighborhood" were allowed in labor and delivery rooms. All felt that families mainly "got in the way" during labor.

70. Fullerton, *Handbook of Obstetric Nursing,* 110.

71. Bernice Gardner, "Nursing Care During the Administration of Rectal Anesthesia," *AJN* 31 (July 1921): 794–98; Anne Yelton and Marie Hilgediek, "Rectal Ether Analgesia from the Nurse's Standpoint," *AJN* 33 (May 1933): 420–22; Harold Rosenfield, "Analgesia in Obstetrics," *AJN* 35 (May 1935): 437–40; Catherine Yeo, "Technic of Administration [Analgesia in Obstetrics] and Nursing Care," *AJN* 35 (May 1935): 440–42; Sandelowski, *Pain, Pleasure and American Childbirth.*

72. Judith Leavitt, "Strange Young Women on Errands."

73. Bland interview.

74. Wertz and Wertz, *Lying-In;* Sandelowski, *Pain, Pleasure and American Childbirth;* and Sylvia Hoffert, *Private Matters: American Attitudes Toward Childbearing and Infant Nurture in the Urban, Ill. North, 1800–1860* (Urbana, Ill.: University of Illinois Press, 1989).

75. Leavitt, "'The Greatest Blessing of This Age': Pain Relief in Obstetrics," in *Brought to Bed.*

76. Mary Blackwell, "The Nursing Care of Obstetric Patients Having Analgesia and Anesthesia," *AJN* 33 (May 1933): 425–27; Pierce Rucker, "Obstetric Analgesia and Anesthesia, " *AJN* 33 (May 1933): 423–25.

77. Sandelowski, *Pain, Pleasure, and American Childbirth,* 68.

78. Anne interview.

79. Charles Rosenberg, *The Care of Strangers* (New York: Basic Books, 1987); Stevens, *In Sickness and in Wealth.*

80. Chelly Wasserberg and Ethel Northam, "Some Time Studies in Obstetrical Nursing," *AJN* 27 (July 1927): 543–44; S. Lillian Clayton, "Standardizing Nursing Technic: Its Advantages and Disadvantages," *AJN* 27 (November 1927): 939–43.

81. Quoted in Mary Louise Habel and Hazel Milton, *The Graduate Nurse in the Home* (Philadelphia: J. B. Lippincott, 1939), 6. These standards were named for Isabel Stewart, who was recognized in 1937 by the National League for Nursing Education (NLNE) for her 25 continuous years of service as Chairman of the Curriculum Committee. The Committee on Curriculum, *Curriculum Guide for Schools of Nursing* (New York: National League for Nursing Education, 1937), v.

82. Nellie Brown, "A Movable Perineal Dressing Tray," *AJN* 24 (November 1924): 875–76; Mildred Newton, "The Noiseless Perineal Dressing Cart," *AJN* 28 (July 1928): 667–68; M. Cordelia Cowen, "A Study of Breast Care: Part I," *AJN* 29 (October 1929): 1165–70; Cowen, "A Study of Breast Care: Part II," *AJN* 29 (November 1929): 1299–1306; DeLee, *Obstetrics for Nurses;* Weeks-Shaw, *Textbook of Nursing;* Louise Zabriskie, *Nurses Handbook of Obstetrics,* 1st through 6th eds. (Philadelphia: J.B. Lippincott, 1929, 1931, 1933, 1934, 1937, and 1940); Carolyn Van Blarcom, *Obstetrical Nursing,* 2nd ed. (New York: Macmillan, 1932).

83. Emily Shaffer, "Perineal Technic," *AJN* 34 (January 1934): 26–28; "A Survey of Methods Used in Four Hospitals," *AJN* 31 (March 1931): 313–17; Joyce Roberts, "Maternal Positions for Childbirth: A Historical Review of Nursing Care Practices," *Journal of Obstetric, Gynecologic, and Neonatal Nursing* 8 (January/February 1979): 24–32.

84. Van Blarcom, *Obstetrical Nursing,* 433.

85. Ibid., 439.

86. Pope, "Obstetric Nursing," 166.

87. Keith, " Preliminaries of Obstetric Nursing, " 259.

88. Hampton, *Nursing,* 379; Worcester, *Monthly Nursng,* 1–10.

89. Lillian, M. (R.N., 1948 graduate Virginia Baptist Hospital), interview by the author, Lynchburg, Va., 24 March 1994.

90. Carolyn L. (R.N., 1933 graduate of Riverside Hospital), *Newport News,* interview by the author, Richmond, Va., 10 March 1993.

91. Jane McLaughlin, "Teaching Obstetrics to Nurses," *AJN* 28 (June 1928): 605–7. Quote is on p. 607.

92. Van Blarcom, *Obstetrical Nursing,* 255.

93. Ibid., 9.

94. Eva Renwick, "Why I Prefer Obstetrics in Private Nursing," *AJN* 17 (October 1916): 42–44. Quote is on p. 43.

95. Van Blarcom, *Obstetrical Nursing,* 11.

96. Ibid., 5.

97. Mary H. (1930 graduate of Stuart Circle Hospital, Richmond,Va.), interview by the author, Lynchburg, Va., 27 April 1994.

98. Historian Patricia O'Brien D'Antonio has urged the recognition of nurses' domestic abilities as the source of their strength and power. Patricia O'Brien D'Antonio, "The Legacy of Domesticity: Nursing in Nineteenth Century America," *Nursing History Review* 1 *(1993)*: 229–46.

99. The intrinsic "fitness" of female nurses providing a womanly service to meet childbearing women's needs was hailed by physicians, nurses, and the public. A physician wrote that the primary qualification for the obstetric nurse, her "most precious characteristic," was her "maternal motherly love for the helpless." Worcester, *Monthly Nursing,* 23. Obstetric nurses listed as valuable attributes traits that were also

associated with womanhood: adaptability, tact, sense of humor, virtue, conscience, courage, alertness of mind, deftness of hand, and "the love of a baby in her heart." Burttle, "*Obstetrical Nursing,*"196. Van Blarcom wrote, "the sympathetic insight which should constantly underlie the work of the obstetric nurse . . . is almost her test as a nurse and a womanly woman, for she needs to be both, supremely." Van Blarcom, *Obstetrical Nursing,* 231. The public press also praised the womanly qualities of nurses. In 1915, Sarah Canstock enthused: "There is something about a nurse—a real one—that makes the rest of us women jealous. . . . She seems to be a sort of embodied womanhood to the *n*th power. Sarah Constock, "Your Daughter's Career," *Good Housekeeping* 61 (December 1915): 728–36.

100. Thomas Olson, "Laying Claim to Caring: Nursing and the Language of Training," *Nursing Outlook* 41 (March/April 1993): 68–72.

101. A. Wilcox, L. Kobayashi, and Murray, "Twenty-five years of obstetric patient satisfaction in North America: A Review of the Literature," *Journal of Perinatal and Neonatal Nursing* 10 (March 1997): 361–78; Brigitte Jordan, *Birth in Four Cultures,* 4th ed. (Prospect Heights: Waveland Press, 1993); Robbie Davis-Floyd, *Birth as an American Rite of Passage* (Berkeley: University of California, 1992); Eakins, *The American Way of Birth.*

102. Linda Kobert, "Are Universal Precautions Changing the 'Nurture' of Obstetric Nursing?" *AJN* 89 (December 1989): 1609. Margarete Sandelowski has conducted extensive investigations into questions about the historical effects of technology on nursing care. See Sandelowski, "(Ir)Reconcilable Differences? The Debate Concerning Nursing and Technology," *Image* 29 (Second Quarter 1997): 169–74; and "Making the Best of Things: Technology in American Nursing, 1870–1940," *Nursing History Review* 5 (1997): 3–22.

103. Joan Lynaugh and Claire Fagin, "Nursing comes of Age," *Image* 20 (Winter 1988): 184–90.

We Must Have Nurses
Spanish Influenza in America 1918–1919

RHONDA KEEN-PAYNE

Harris College of Nursing
Texas Christian University

Heralded as the Spanish Lady, she emptied church pews, school desks, and pool halls. She killed soldiers in trenches in France far more efficiently than any shell or mustard gas. For 10 months the Spanish Lady danced with partners around the world. She then disappeared as mysteriously as she came and was even more quickly forgotten.

Against the backdrop of the deadly monotonous stalemate of World War I, an influenza type A virus was traveling through the populations of the world at speeds far in excess of a soldier's march, although the virus would certainly hitch a ride with him when possible. The virus was generous in its visitation, effective in its infestation, and accurate in its aim.

In the 1920s estimates suggested that the flu killed at least twenty-two million people within 10 months.[1] More recent analyses indicate that this estimate of mortality is quite low because data from large parts of China and Africa, were not included.[2] The combined battle deaths of American soldiers in World Wars 1 and 2, Korea, and Vietnam total 423,000 compared to the certainly low estimate of 675,000 Americans felled by the flu in 1918. Not only was this virus deadly, but it displayed an affinity for mortality much like war, striking young adults in the prime of life as often as elders and babies.[3]

Nevertheless, students of American history asked to name significant events of the 20th century are unlikely to recall this devastating illness. Likewise, American history textbooks written by the most thorough of authors may devote a page or two to the epidemic. Instead historians of the 20th century focus on topics such as politics, domestic and international policies related to economic and foreign affairs, and, of course, war.

Nursing History Review 8 (2000): 143-156. A publication of the American Association for the History of Nursing. Copyright © 2000 Springer Publishing Company.

The effects of the flu were further obscured by the actions of organized medicine. The young profession responded to the critical 1910 report by Abraham Flexner in a variety of ways, including a tendency to guard its history. As medicine increased its social status, it increasingly portrayed itself as a discipline that could only be understood by those with a background in laboratory science. Thus, possible historians were discouraged from further exploration into topics related to science, medicine, health, or illness.[4]

Occurrences such as the 1918 influenza pandemic offer an opportunity to understand the integration of personal and family life, healthcare and policy, and biology within the context of the crisis. Pandemics shake the foundations of society and offer for examination a cross-section of values, assumptions, and practices of the whole society. Historian Charles Rosenberg summarized the value of an epidemic for social studies as "an extraordinarily useful sampling device."[5]

Epidemiology

The term epidemic describes a singular event, dramatic and public, which is immediately visible to contemporary observers.[6] An epidemic also conveys expectations of a significant degree of morbidity and mortality and of geographic spread. Pandemic is used to describe epidemics with total world spread and is synonymous with epidemics of great proportions. Characteristic behaviors of an influenza epidemic include sudden onset, dispersion throughout an area within a month, and then dispersion throughout the continent of origin and the world in a few months. Influenza epidemics affect people of all economic and social levels and those of every age. It has a high morbidity but a fairly low mortality rate, with most deaths among the old or those with chronic illnesses.[7]

Other influenza pandemics can be identified from historical review: at least three in the 19th century, followed by one in 1918, another in 1957, and the most recent in 1968. Epidemics are currently named for the area in which the virus is first isolated. Historically, geographic names were attached to epidemics according to the area first or most associated with the outbreak of infection. Hence, the 1918 virus was labeled Spanish influenza or, more familiarly, the Spanish Lady. Although the infection most certainly did not begin in Spain, it was widely publicized there. The king of Spain was ill with the virus. Spain did not black out news during the war, therefore, information about its epidemic was released to the press.[8]

There are concerns about the reliability of data sources with regard to the 1918 flu that exceed the normal problems of historical evidence. First, the countries at war, including the United States, were under news blackouts at least part of the time, and several of the governments involved actively censored and controlled the press releases of the day. The United States, entering the war late and against the German front, was cautious in releasing the morbidity and mortality statistics of flu victims, especially those of soldiers or in areas where major military installations were located. Second, some news reports may have deliberately painted a brighter picture than was accurate. Beyond merely suppressing negative reports, the purpose of such reporting was to mislead the enemy and encourage one's allies. Third, the isolation of rural and remote areas contributed to a significant lack of information gathered and recorded. As much as 22% of the United States population lived in areas that were not a part of the vital statistics record-keeping system at the time.[9] Data related to health, even simple demographic information such as births and deaths, were not collected. Last, some areas were interested in bolstering their images for reasons unrelated to the war and may have failed to report or reported falsely low morbidity and mortality data. Atlanta, for example, was known at the time for its boosterism and self-promotion efforts to attract business investments. For all these reasons, when the significance of the flu epidemic is considered, data should be interpreted as conservative in the extreme.

Health and Healthcare in the United States

The 1918 influenza epidemic struck at a time when the outlook for public health had never been brighter. Multiple medical and scientific advances were made in the late 19th and early 20th centuries. In 1884, Robert Koch identified the steps for establishing causation between an organism and disease while studying tuberculosis.[10] Using Koch's method, the causative microorganisms of malaria, typhoid, tetanus, tuberculosis, and diphtheria were identified. The virus eluded study because it was so small that it passed through the porcelain filters that snagged bacteria, but its presence was suspected. A mosquito was discovered as the vector for yellow fever in Cuba, and Salvarsan was identified as a treatment for syphilis. The identification of blood groups, improvements in surgery and maternal-infant care, and isolation of the thyroid hormone soon followed. The first vitamin was discovered in 1911.[11]

Physicians and their control of the profession underwent rapid change in the first 2 decades of the 20th century. Several studies had indicated the need for educational and professional reform, and after Hexner's 1910 recommendations, many philanthropic foundations funded schools of medicine and research as well as hospitals to support the improved medical practice of the period. In general, medicine and physicians as professional practitioners were gaining in stature and power in the community throughout the progressive era.[12]

At the same time, organized nursing was taking similar if less dramatic steps to establish control over practice via the registration movement. Lacking funding and social power, nursing leaders faced a more complex professional reform future. Significant strides were made but were made slowly. The Army and Navy Nurse Corps were established. The nurses at the Henry Street Settlement House brought dramatic attention to the health and lives of immigrants, and nurses found a home in the sanitation movement. [13]

Nurses, physicians, and other public health reformers had cause for pride. With the application of findings from the laboratory a variety of public health protective measures were instituted. The battle against tuberculosis, the Great White Plague, was certainly taken over by these groups. They encouraged various state legislatures and medical schools to educate the public on preventive measures to arrest the spread of the disease. A pure milk campaign was added to prevention efforts. The milk campaign was a part of the food and drug legislation proposed to protect the public from impurities and contamination. A variety of other advances, including vaccinations and inoculations, were supported by organized nursing, medicine, and public health reform leaders. [14]

The American Public Health Association (APHA) led a campaign for legislation to insure that vital statistics would be collected by every state on birth and death. Prior to this one historian noted, some states' records of human statistics were less adequate than those for terrapins, oysters, and pedigreed stock.[15] By 1913, 22 states were within compliance of the census requirements, more than double the number in 1901.

Public health advances were numerous, but none would have any practical impact on the management of influenza. Prevention, treatment, and containment were largely ineffective against a loafing organism with the ability to change as its hosts became immune. The virus struck in the spring of 1918, shifted its genetic form, returned for a second deadly episode in early autumn, and then circled the globe a final time after Armistice Day.

Nature and Charcteristics of Influenza Type A

Influenza continues to be among the top ten killers of Americans and is suspected to have existed for many generations. It is caused by a virus, one of the smallest microorganisms, which is characterized by the nature of its reproduction. The virus takes over the host cell's building blocks and mechanisms for its own replication. There are three types of influenza viruses, but only type A is related to the 1918 epidemic.

The structure of the influenza type A virus explains a great deal about the nature of the disease of influenza. The spherical surface, approximately 1/10,000 millimeter in diameter, is covered with spiking protrusions. Its appearance is that of a dandelion with stiff rather than billowy spikes. These spikes are antigens, material that stimulates the virus's host to develop antibodies for protection. Although two other antigens are contained within the virus's membrane, the surface antigens are key to the nature of the virus. All type A viruses have two surface antigens; they are hemagglutinin (H), which causes red blood cells to clump, and neuraminidase (N), an enzyme.[16]

The H and N antigens are unique and are numerically identified; thus, the virus responsible for the 1968 Hong Kong influenza was an H3, N2 subtype. The virus subtype in the 1918 pandemic has been identified, by the presence of antibodies isolated from persons who survived the infection, as a probable H1, N1 subtype.[17]

Each combination of different antigens represents a new subtype of the virus. If the H and N antigens change only marginally, antigenic *drift* has occurred. A degree of host immunity remains because the host's antibodies continue to recognize sufficient features of the virus. A mild outbreak or limited epidemic may be observed.

More dramatic alterations in the H and N antigens are called antigenic *shifts*. The result is a new combination of antigens for which potential hosts have no immunity because the host has no circulating antibodies that recognize the new H and N antigens. When antigenic shift occurs, a subtype capable of causing pandemic influenza exists.[18]

Edwin Kilbourne described the growth of an epidemic as an event that smolders before it bursts into flames.[19] This is probably explained by the virus's antigenic drift and shift, by patterns of travel, and, possibly, by a seasonal influence on the virus's growth and transmission. In general, hosts are protected by antibodies from each virus they encounter. As viruses experience antigenic shifts and drifts, the original virus is eliminated, and repetitions of the same virus are unlikely.

Equally important to understanding epidemic influenza is an appreciation of the similarity of viruses found in humans and animals. Type A influenza viruses have been isolated in birds, swine, horses, and other fowl.[20] Some researchers believe that many influenza epidemics in humans have their origins in China because large populations of ducks and other fowl are found there living in close contact with humans. The H1, N1 influenza of 1918 is believed to have originated in birds. Research conducted on ribonucleic acid (RNA) fragments indicated that the virus altered its form as it passed through the swine population and possibly mixed with swine viruses. It then entered the human population with a new and particularly potent antigenic combination.[21]

The virus is transmitted by droplet contamination. The route may be indirect, via sneezing and coughing, as well as direct, via kissing or sharing eating utensils. The incubation period, the time from infection to symptoms, is quite short, ranging from 1 to 3 days.

Influenza, including the 1918 infection, is manifested by a sudden onset, hence the English nickname of "knock-me-down-fever." In 1918 the symptoms included a fever that lasted from 3 to 5 days, punctuated by severe chilling; a dry, burning throat and hacking cough accompanied headache and muscle aches in the limbs and back; and once the fever subsided, a watery nasal discharge followed, and in serious cases, a severe nosebleed. Survivors experienced general weakness, fatigue, and depression that lasted another few weeks.

The most serious complication was pneumonia, "influenza's colleague in death."[22] It usually occurs in about 20% of all influenza cases. In 1918 the incidence was much more common, and the cases were more complicated. Pneumonia was characterized by pulmonary hemorrhages and an abundant discharge that compromised breathing. The lungs of the sickest victims seemed to be overflowing with bloody fluid. At this stage most were cyanotic, their skin described as blue and even purple. Some nurses reportedly used the color of the feet in triage decisions; those with black feet would not live.[23]

The First Wave

The flu struck in three waves. The first wave was relatively unremarkable, only a hint of what was to come. The first cases of influenza and pneumonia were reported in March 1918; soldiers in stateside camps as well as those arriving in Europe were sick. By mid-May the epidemic was entrenched alongside the soldiers in both America and Europe. It was reported in every army and in towns and cities in England, France, Belgium, Germany, Russia, and the United States.[24] As entire fleets and armies were infected, resources that would have been poured into offensive actions were instead directed toward the nursing or burial of soldiers. Obviously, soldiers prostrated with fulminating infection were unable to perform. In the United States a draft was canceled; in Germany the failure of a significant July offensive was blamed on the poor condition of the German soldiers.[25]

Likewise, the war influenced the infection. The intimate relationship between enthusiastic crowds and droplet-borne infection was never so apparent as on 12 September 1918. Just as the lethal second wave began, thirteen million men lined up to register for the draft. Alfred Crosby called this interweaving of war and pandemic "a pattern of complete insanity."[26]

The first wave lasted to midsummer, and influenza deaths were recorded in China, North Africa, New Zealand, and India. Although certainly milder than the second wave, the pattern of the virus was established with the first infections and deaths. The symptoms were characteristic, with two notable exceptions. More people than usual were dying of this flu, and the death rate was unusually high in young adults, aged twenty to forty. As the first wave waned, killing tens of thousands, the fall onslaught was quietly beginning.

The Second Wave

The influenza type A virus had probably undergone an antigenic shift in either China or the United States that increased its already deadly virulence by late August. The second wave of the flu and accompanying pneumonia killed millions of people worldwide before Armistice Day.

The flu traveled across America along the pathways of ordinary transportation, from east to west. Although never routinely predictable, there was a general pattern of infection, which followed the highways, railroad tracks, and shipping lanes. Some isolated rural areas were missed altogether. Most crowded urban areas were devastated quickly, with the incidence of infectious cases dwindling as quickly as it had accelerated.

The effects of the pandemic are most apparent in urban areas. Pandemic influenza induces fear, as does any plague, but it strikes quickly; action and response are demanded. The massive infection crippled systems of government, health care, and social services and overwhelmed every support service and facility involved as well as individual nurses, physicians, and volunteers who worked as long as they could stand. The horror and grief of widespread death was mixed with the irritating frustration of daily inconvenience.

In response to the second wave the United States Public Health Service (USPHS) launched an information campaign in September explaining the flu and asking for volunteers to assist the medical corps. Eventually, over 72,000 physicians volunteered to back up the USPHS. At the same time, 1500 nurses volunteered through the Red Cross in Washington, D.C., alone.[27] However, as everyone soon learned, there simply were not enough nurses to go around. The nurse in Katherine Anne Porter's *Pale Horse Pale Rider* remarked "Nursing is nine-tenths, just the same," and so it was; nursing care of warmth, rest, and fluids was the only intervention.[28]

In most cities, local health departments were assisted by the USPHS in educating citizens, and thousands of posters and placards were distributed. In Newark, persons were advised to dress warmly, avoid crowds, cover mouth and nose when sneezing, and go to bed at the earliest sign of illness.[29] At the same time, however, the events of the war countermanded the health department bulletins. Ten days after the Bureau of Health had issued its warning, the Fourth Liberty Loan Drive was kicked off in Philadelphia with a parade that stretched twenty-three blocks and drew 200,000 spectators. Liberty bonds were bought in record numbers.[30] Four weeks later, 7,800 residents of Philadelphia were dead of the flu and pneumonia.[31]

Contagion control was addressed in a variety of ways. In Chicago, persons who sneezed openly or who spit were threatened with arrests and fines. Churches were not closed, but parishioners were requested to stay home if ill, and windows were opened for ventilation during services. By the third week in October, the peak of the second wave, closings had extended to theaters, banquets, lectures, restaurants, and movie shows.[32]

In Newark the state simply banned all public gatherings on 10 October. Although some civic leaders feared that the ban would cause panic, cooperation was relatively widespread for a week. Confusion developed when liquor stores were allowed to remain open for sales, although not for congregating. Many church leaders protested the ban as detrimental to the morale of the citizens and cited the liquor store exemption. The ban was lifted 21 October, but not before some politicians had been damaged by their support of liquor stores.[33]

San Diego's board of health closed all public facilities, which included libraries, pool halls, women's weekly club meetings, and all outdoor meetings except those convened to sell Liberty Loan bonds. The ban was lifted and then imposed again as new cases of influenza increased; citizens were never strongly supportive of the measures.

Many cities also required that masks be worn in public. These were most often fashioned of several layers of square gauze and tied at the top of the head and behind the neck. Some were sprayed with various disinfectants. In some areas the masks were religiously worn; compliance in others, however, was spotty. In San Diego an editorial in the *San Diego Union* lampooned the masks, complaining that pretty faces were obscured, that the colors should be red, white, and blue, and that only burglars wore masks professionally.[34]

The breakdown in social systems had an effect on the ordinary, mundane activities of daily living: telephone companies were unable to handle more than emergency calls; public transportation was interrupted as train and taxi operators fell ill; and food shortages were caused by sickness on the farm or at the shop. Essential services were threatened as well. Nurses and other health workers were absent or sick themselves; firefighters and police officers were unable to work; and teachers and priests left their students and parishioners without guidance. Families were struck randomly, both by disease and death, and the flu killed the usual survivors, the young adults in their prime, disproportionately more often than others.

Two examples of collapse in services are noteworthy. First, the overwhelming demand for nursing and hospital services outstripped the supply within a week of the onset of the first cases. In Cleveland the Visiting Nurse Association had an increase of 400% in their caseload in a week. In their annual report for the year the association noted shortages of nurses and "intelligent relatives."[35] Particularly in large cities with crowded immigrant tenements, nurses and doctors worked as many hours and for as many days as they could stand upright. Most anecdotes describe 18-hour days as the usual course during the peak of the second wave. Lillian Wald, founder of public health nursing in New York City, wrote to a friend that "the wolf is scratching at our door" in explaining that 40,000 nurses were needed for the city's poor.[36]

Hospitals in Newark were completely overwhelmed with civilians as well as soldiers from nearby bases. The county system was willing to provide space but required the city to send its own nurses and doctors, the commodity in shortest supply everywhere. The city finally purchased a warehouse and set up 400 beds that were staffed with a thin pool of volunteer doctors and nurses. Women with any training at all in care of the ill were recruited. Eventually, the crisis passed, enabled by the Red Cross which coordinated the volunteer efforts of about 200 women from the ranks of Roman Catholic sisterhoods, student nurses, and other volunteer groups.[37]

The experience of public health nurses varied across the nation. In Philadelphia they found themselves taxed at every step to visit families sick with the flu. In other areas, nurses were shunned for fear they might be contagious. In San Francisco a crisis was quickly under way before the flu had even peaked. The Red Cross reported that it could meet only half the demand placed on its services. Thousands of volunteers, medical and nursing students, teachers idled because of closed schools, priests and nuns, and finally, the general public came to the aid of sick San Franciscans.[38]

The need for nurses in rural areas and small towns is not well documented. A few anecdotes are published in 1919 issues of the *American Journal of Nursing* and *Public Health Nursing*. One nurse wrote of her experience in a northern Michigan logging camp. Upon her arrival at the camp she found nearly everyone sick and piled into one-room cabins together. She was especially concerned about the practice of spitting without regard to contagion; the nurse finally managed to control some of the risk by providing a tin can on a chair beside each bed. She instructed adult women in care and visited often; the mortality was restricted to one infant death.[39]

Two other accounts of nurses in rural areas offer different perspectives. In a small town in North Dakota, nurses had to milk cows and launder linens for families they found ill.[40] Beulah Gribble was called to nurse at a coal mining camp in Kentucky where she estimated 1,000 of 2,500 residents were ill. Neighbors assisted each other, providing minimal care and food. Only one doctor was available, and many families lived in remote areas. The local recreation building was converted to a hospital, and the sickest patients were seen there.[41]

Most nurses wanted assistance in knowing how to handle the epidemic's contagion as well as recommendations regarding the care of patients. A report was issued by the USPHS's Committee on Administrative Measures for Relief in the *American Journal of Nursing* that offered guidelines for nurses. The report was specific and practical, with sections on food and laundry management, patient and community education, and provisions for care of the dead. Unfortunately, its usefulness in the epidemic was negligible because it was not published until the mild third wave was ending.[42]

In all, nursing and medical care suffered greatly because of shortages due first to the war but mostly due to the tremendous demand of cases. In retrospect, however, most care needed was simple and could have been provided by anyone with minimal instruction from the nurses or doctors. The worst cases were those in isolated areas where entire families were stricken or in crowded slums with no resources for support.

Burying the Dead

Even more challenging, according to some reports, was the strain on morgues and burial facilities and processes. The dead accumulated faster than any undertaker could manage, and the system was stressed from the point of picking up dead bodies to shoveling dirt over caskets. Crosby reported the chilling advice offered from the East Coast to the rest of the nation: "Hunt up your woodworkers and cabinetmakers and set them to making coffins."[43] The advice concluded with instructions to begin grave digging in preparation for the wave of mortality that was headed west. In Philadelphia, bodies accumulated rapidly in the third week of October. The city morgue had several hundred bodies in a space designed for thirty-six. Most were not embalmed, and there was no ice. The city government took over, transported bodies to a cold storage plant, and turned to several local woodworking companies. Within two weeks, 2,100 coffins had been produced at a charge of 20% above production costs. Part of the contract stipulated that the coffins were to be used to bury only residents of Philadelphia.[44]

Disposal of bodies was a problem in many urban and rural areas. In Buffalo the city produced its own coffins. In Washington a health officer reportedly commandeered two railroad cars of coffins headed for Philadelphia.[45] In an isolated community in the Ozark mountains a farmer enlisted the aid of two neighbors to help him carry the bodies of his two sons, both in their early twenties, across a suspension footbridge to a mountain cemetery. Upon reaching the cemetery the farmer opened the coffin lids in order to make final arrangements to his sons' bodies. His neighbors fled, fearing contamination, and he was left to dig both graves alone.[46]

As much as the contamination threat of decaying corpses, the sight of unburied bodies is a serious threat to the morale of a community. Body preparation rituals are important to many cultures, and no American families were satisfied leaving their dead where they fell. The imperative felt by local officials to manage bodies was probably not out of proportion to the importance of the problem.

Aftermath

The second wave, by far the most deadly, peaked in most American cities before Armistice Day. The third and final wave, hardly perceived in some areas, was completed by late winter in some areas and by late spring by nearly all. The Spanish Lady left, essentially, with the war.

Approximately one-fourth of the American population fell ill with influenza in 1918—1919, and at least 675,000 died of the flu and pneumonia. In addition to the limitations of reported data noted earlier, also omitted from mortality reports are those who died of complications of chronic illnesses made worse by the flu, or those who died of other acute disorders related to the flu, such as bronchitis.[47]

Among those who died were the usual age groups of the very young and very old but also those aged twenty to forty. An explanation for this unusual peak in mortality has not been found. Immigrants and the poor also died disproportionately more frequently than their native born, wealthier fellows. There are several possible explanations, but none confirmed, including genetic differences, exposure and immunity, or associated factors such as nutritional status.[48]

The influenza epidemic also cost the nation in economic terms, although no satisfactory estimate exists. The cost included such factors as insurance payments, work lost, services and systems interrupted temporarily or permanently, and the loss of productive adults to the work force.

Other costs, of course, of emotional energy and morale are even more difficult to measure. Memory of the event does not seem to extend beyond the generation who experienced the epidemic, but the memories of this group are profound. Elsie Kathryn Laura Schlierer was married on her twenty-first birthday, 10 October 1918, to Emil Schermeister in Philadelphia. Neither of them felt well during the wedding, and they were put to bed afterward in separate rooms. By the time she wakened the following day, she was a widow. She recovered from the flu, lived a long, rewarding life, but for a few years in her twenties, she was the Widow Schermeister.[49]

Finally, the mystery of the absence of the flu in our memories bears mention. Crosby suggested that no real mystery exists. After all, epidemics had come and gone before, no one famous died, and it lasted only 10 months. Most important, though, was the larger-than-life war in Europe, the carnage of the century that reduced everything else to trivia.[50] The flu, for many and perhaps for most, was only one more grim component of an already dreadful war.

RHONDA KEEN-PAYNE, RN, PhD
Harris College of Nursing
Texas Christian University
110 Walters Lane
Weatherford, TX 76087

Notes

1. Edwin Oakes Jordan, *Epidemic Influenza, A Survey* (Chicago: American Medical Association, 1927), 214–18. Most modern epidemiological methods now indicate much higher morbidity and mortality figures.

2. K. David Patterson, *Pandemic Influenza, 1700–1900* (Totawa, N.J.: Rowman & Littlefield, Publishers, 1986), 1.

3. Alfred W. Crosby, *Epidemic and Peace, 1918* (Westport, Conn.: Greenwood Press, 1976), 206–7. Crosby's work continues to be the definitive reference; for contemporaneous data, see also W.H. Frost, *Public Health Reports, 35* (1920): 584.

4. Charles E. Rosenberg, *Explaining Epidemics and Other Studies in the History of Medicine* (New York: Cambridge University Press, 1992), 2.

5. Ibid., 279.

6. Ibid., 279.

7. W. I. B. Beveridge, *Influenza: The Last Great Plague: An Unfinished Story of Discovery* (New York: Prodist, 1977), 18.

8. This infection has a variety of names but is most often called the flu. Although the epidemic lasted from March 1918 through early summer 1919, it is most often referred to as the 1918 flu because the vast majority of morbidity and mortality occurred in the fall of 1918.

9. Crosby, *Epidemic and Peace,* 206.

10. Thomas Brock, *Milestones in Microbiology* (Englewood Cliffs, N.J.: Prentice-Hall, 1961), 116–17.

11. Charles Singer and E. Ashworth Underwood, *A Short History of Medicine* (New York: Oxford University Press, 1962), 612, 637; Edwin H. Ackerknecht, *A Short History of Medicine* (New York: Ronald Press Co., 1955), 213.

12. James G. Burrow, *Organized Medicine in the Progressive Era* (Baltimore: Johns Hopkins University Press, 1977), 12.

13. Philip A. Kalisch and Beatrice J. Kalisch, *The Advance of American Nursing,* 3rd ed. (Boston: Little, Brown, and Co., 1995), 171–210.

14. Burrow, *Organized Medicine,* 88–102; Kalisch and Kalisch, *Advance of American Nursing,* 124–56.

15. Burrow, *Organized Medicine,* 99.

16. Edward Alcamo, *Fundamentals of Microbiology,* 4th ed. (Redwood City, Calif.: Benjamin/Cummings Publishing Co., 1994), 327–39.

17. Jeffrey Taubenberger et al., "Initial Genetic Characterization of the 1918 'Spanish' Influenza Virus," *Science 275,* (March 1997): 1793–96.

18. Beveridge, *Influenza,* 70–73.

19. Edwin D. Kilbourne, ed., *The Influenza Viruses and Influenza* (New York: Academic Press, 1975).

20. Ibid.; Patterson, *Pandemic Influenza,* 4–5, 84–85.

21. Taubenberger, "Initial Genetic Characterization," 1795.

22. Kalisch, *Advance of American Nursing,* 360.

23. Malcolm Gladwell, "The Dead Zone," *The New Yorker,* 29 September 1997, 55. This is an account of the beginning of the partial exhumation of six Norwegian miners, flu victims buried in the permafrost; Kirsty Duncan lead the autopsy team, hoping to recover genetic fragments of the 1918 virus in the form of RNA residue. Several articles about the flu have recently appeared in popular literature, including *The New York Times Magazine* and *Rolling Stone.*

24. Crosby, *Epidemic and Peace,* 21–26.

25. Crosby, *Epidemic and Peace,* 49; Erich von Ludendorff, *Ludendorff's Own Story* (New York: Harper and Brothers, 1919), 2: 277, 317.

26. Crosby, *Epidemic and Peace,* 51.

27. Crosby, *Epidemic and Peace*, 46.

28. Katherine Anne Porter, *Pale Horse, Pale Rider* (New York: Harcourt, Brace, and World, 1936), 161. Her classic short novel tells the story of a young couple in San Francisco both ill with the flu; she recovers to find him dead. The title is taken from the American spiritual "Pale horse, pale rider, Done taken my lover away." from Rev. 6:8.

29. Stuart Galishoff, "Newark and the Great Influenza Pandemic of 1918," *New England Journal of Medicine* 64 (n.d.): 249.

30. Crosby, *Epidemic and Peace*, 72.

31. Ibid.

32. Paul A. Buelow, "Chicago," in *The 1918–1919 Pandemic of Influenza: The Urban Impact in the Western World*, ed. Fred R. van Hartesveldt (Lewiston, N.Y.: Edwin Mellen Press, 1992), 132–38.

33. Galishoff, *Newark and the Great Influenza Pandemic*, 251–55.

34. *San Diego Union*, Oct. 21, 1918, as quoted by Richard Peterson, "San Diego" in van Hartesveldt, ed., *1918–1919 Pandemic*, 152.

35. Buelow, "Chicago," 143.

36. Beth Siegel, *Lillian Wald of Henry Street* (New York: Macmillan, 1983), 146.

37. Galishoff, *Newark and the Great Influenza Pandemic*, 251–54.

38. Crosby, *Epidemic and Peace*, 76, 92–97.

39. Ann Colon, "Experiences During the Epidemic Influenza at Cedar Branch Camp," *American Journal of Nursing* 19 (October 1919): 605–7.

40. R.G. "Experiences during the Influenza Epidemic," *American Journal of Nursing* 19 (March 1919): 203–4.

41. Beulah Gribble, "Experiences during the Epidemic: Influenza in a Kentucky Coal-Mining Camp," *American Journal of Nursing* 19, no. (August 1919): 609–11.

42. E. Foley, "Department of Public Health Nursing," *American Journal of Nursing* 19, (May 1919): 377–82.

43. Crosby, *Epidemic and Peace*, 92.

44. Ibid., 82–83.

45.   Ibid.

46. Mrs. Emma Hoskins Holland, interview by author, tape recording, Fayetteville, Ark., 18 October 1996. She is the younger sister of the two brothers who died; the flu killed several young men in the isolated Ozark mountain community of Aurora, Arkansas. There were no doctors or nurses in the area.

47. Crosby, *Epidemic and Peace*, 203–7.

48. Ibid., 229–55.

49. She lived 98 years. Dr. Rose Cannon, personal communication to the author, 25 September 1998, recalling her mother's memories of the flu in Philadelphia. In Porter's heroine's words, "No more war, no more plague, only the dazed silence that follows the ceasing of heavy guns; noiseless houses with the shades drawn, empty streets, the dead cold light of tomorrow. Now there would be time for everything."

50. Suggested by this rhyme chant for jumping rope, "I had a little bird And its name was Enza. I opened the window And In-Flew-Enza." Crosby, *Epidemic and Peace*, 319–25.

The Miners' Hospitals of West Virginia
Nurses and Healthcare Come to the Coal Fields, 1900–1920

JOHN C. KIRCHGESSNER
School of Nursing
University of Virginia

Industrialization during the last quarter of the 19th century brought incredible changes in the state of West Virginia. The timber and railroad industries paved the way for the most influential industry of all, coal mining. The coal industry began in West Virginia in the late 1870s and remained strong for over 80 years. During this 80-year period the state of West Virginia was changed forever. Industrialization changed all aspects of life, including healthcare. The local physicians and the coal company doctors could not manage the trauma and surgical patients that were coming to them from the coal fields. In response, the state of West Virginia created three hospitals dedicated to the care of those employees injured as a result of their employment.

This article is part of an ongoing study focusing on the healthcare in the West Virginia coal fields and three miners' hospitals. Here I try to explain why and how the miners' hospitals were established. Next, I argue that in spite of horrendous occupational injuries and social conditions, nurses and physicians working in these hospitals managed to improve the outcome of at least some of their patients.

DANGEROUS WORK: EARLY MINING IN WEST VIRGINIA

Work in the mines during the early years of King Coal was hazardous to the miners' lives and limbs. The mines of the late 19th and early 20th centuries varied greatly in their safety. Miners were exposed to occupational hazards such as crushing, burns, and fractures every day of their working lives, with few provisions for accident prevention and medical care. The safety regulations for mining were lax and were not readily enforced.[1] Melody Bragg notes that poor mining conditions were related to the fact that the mines were located in areas

Nursing History Review 8 (2000): 157-168. A publication of the American Association for the History of Nursing. Copyright © 2000 Springer Publishing Company.

to which mining was so new that the dangers that accompanied it were not fully realized or understood. In addition, many of the thousands of men who came to coal mines had never done mining in their lives and had never been trained to deal with the dangers that accompanied underground mining.[2] Miners frequently found themselves lying in water and mud to mine the coal. Coal dust and natural gas were other hazards that miners dealt with on a daily basis. The buildup of natural gas and coal dust not only contributed to the lung ailments that many miners suffered from but also increased the risk of fires and explosions. Rock falls and roof cave-ins were other occupational hazards faced by miners everyday.

During the late 19th and early 20th centuries, electricity and mechanization had not yet come to the mines. Mining was mostly a hand operation with the assistance of animals. In some cases, dogs were used to pull the carts in the smaller and narrower mines where mules and oxen were too tall to maneuver through the passageways. Prior to loading and hauling the coal the miners had to excavate the coal from the seams. This in itself was a task that threatened lives. The method used during this period required the miner to place the explosive black powder, ignite it, and retreat as quickly as possible. Provided that there was not an explosion or fire from the accumulation of gas and coal dust, or a cave-in from the slate roof, the entire process would then be started over again of detaching, shoveling, hauling, and loading the coal. The days were long. The miners usually entered the mines at dawn and finished after sunset, working 12-14 hours a day, 6 days a week.

Child labor laws in the late 19th and early 20th centuries were all but nonexistent, and those that did exist were abided by infrequently.[3] Children who worked in the mines were exposed to the same dangers as the adult miners, and like the adult miners, there was little in the way of compensation for the risks to their health. It was not until 1907 that the state of West Virginia passed legislation prohibiting boys under the age of 14 in the mines; girls were prohibited all together.[4] Coal miners of all ages were subjected to one of the hardest forms of physical labor. Aside from the chronic physical exhaustion these men and boys endured, the risks to their health were innumerable and included acute problems such as burns, fractures, amputations, and lacerations, as well as chronic lung disease and arthritis.

Medical care in the Appalachian Mountains of West Virginia was virtually nonexistent during most of the 19th century. Physicians were few and generally found only in larger towns or cities. The medical care that did exist was usually based on folklore and dispensed by midwives and women in the family. There were, however, nontraditional doctors known as "grannies" or yarb doctors. These local medicine men and women were experts in combining folklore and herbal remedies. Hex doctors also existed and were the equivalent to modern day psychiatrists. As primitive as this form of care may seem, these practitioners and their remedies did try to meet the medical needs of the mountain families.[5,6]

THE MINERS' HOSPITALS

With literally thousands of people coming into the state the few physicians could not meet all of the medical care needs. To provide for the miners and their families, mining companies employed their own physicians. These men were the first to bring modern medicine to the mountains. All were formally trained in medicine, although their training and experience varied. In the coal fields of West Virginia the company doctors had to be self-reliant for there were few resources available other than their own knowledge, experience, and common sense. There were few hospitals, and the ones that did exist were hours away, so the company physicians had to be skilled in both medicine and surgery, often operating in the patients' homes. Some company doctors supervised the healthcare for two or three mining camps. Their work never seemed to cease. Most physicians were on call 24 hours a day in addition to their regularly scheduled office hours and house calls. The quality of care the company physicians provided did vary. In general, however, the company doctors were revered in their communities for their work and the help that they brought to so many families.

The camp physician did not just play the role of the physician but had a variety of healthcare roles. As noted, he was medical doctor and surgeon as well as camp sanitarian. Mine injuries, however, were the greatest challenge to the company doctors. Common injuries included burns, crushed limbs, broken backs, lacerations, and fractured skulls. Often, the surgery required to care for these injuries was done on office exam tables or at home. Chloroform and antiseptics, such as carbolic acid, had been introduced to the coal fields by the early physicians, but major surgery still had a high mortality rate.[7] Few victims survived amputations, spinal trauma, or head trauma. As coal mining expanded in West Virginia and the acuity of the injuries increased, the coal company doctors and the local physicians realized that better medical facilities were needed for the miners and their families, medical care that could not be given in a home or office.[8]

Dr. Henry Hatfield, later West Virginia's Governor Hatfield, initiated efforts to develop regional hospitals in proximity to the coal fields. Hatfield first lobbied the coal mining and railroad companies for financial support.

Neither industry was interested in financing such a venture. Hatfield then lobbied the West Virginia State Legislature. As a result of his persistent efforts the legislature passed a state senate bill, in February 1899, establishing three state-funded miners' hospitals in the coal fields. The hospitals would be for the treatment of "persons injured while engaged in employments dangerous to health, life, and limb."[9] People with infectious diseases would be restricted from admission. Railroad workers, miners, and other laborers injured as a result of their occupations would be admitted and cared for free of charge. Citizens of the region requiring acute care would also be admitted but on a fee for service basis.[10,11] By 1903 the legislature amended the original bill stating that it was the duty of the board of directors of each facility to admit anyone injured or requiring hospitalization.[12] Hospitals were planned for the Flat Top, New River, and Fairmont coal regions and known as Miners' Hospitals No. 1, No. 2, and No. 3, respectively.[13] Other provisions established by the legislature stipulated that each of the hospitals must be convenient to railroad transportation, and each hospital board would be allotted fifteen thousand dollars for construction of the facilities and five thousand dollars annually for maintenance costs.[14,15] Each hospital would have a governor-appointed board of directors consisting of four members, two of whom were from each hospital.[16]

All three hospitals opened their doors to patients in 1901. The story of Miners' Hospital No. 2, later to be known as McKendree Hospital No. 2, represents what nursing and healthcare were like in all of the miners' hospitals. The site of the hospital in McKendree, West Virginia, overlooked the New River Gorge. Joseph Beury, one of the area coal barons, donated the original six and one half acres. Beury was influential in having the hospital placed in the New River Gorge. At the time the town of McKendree was barely more than a village of about fifty citizens, most of whom were lumbermen. While McKendree may have been an idyllic setting, it was isolated and remote.[17] However, the town did have a railroad depot, one of the state requirements for placement of the hospitals, and most of McKendree's patients would arrive by train.[18] Later, as the number of admissions increased, the distance between the depot and hospital became a concern and was remedied by improving the road to the hospital and purchasing an ambulance.

The original hospital was a large two and a half story brick and stone structure, as were Miners' Hospitals No. 1 and No. 3. The grounds also included a few out buildings, such as the stable, icehouse, and shed. The main hospital building contained administrative offices, the superintendent's and staff's home, supply rooms, kitchen, employee's rooms, and the local post office. The staff's homes and employee rooms were racially segregated, as were the patient wards. The patient bed capacity of the hospital was forty-two. Almost immediately after opening, the hospital was filled to capacity. By 1902 the Board of Directors for Hospital No. 2 reported to the West Virginia Board of Control that the capacity of the hospital limited the number of patients that could be treated and further expansion was necessary.[19] Biennial reports from Miners' Hospitals No. 1 and No. 3 reflect similar physical constraints and concerns as the populations in the coal fields continued to grow.[20,21,22] As mining and the state's population continued to expand, the hospitals' superintendents continually asked for more money to expand the facilities. Expansion of Miners' Hospital No. 2, however, would not come until after 1916, when a nurses' home was built.[23] When the nurses' home was completed, the areas of the hospital that previously housed the superintendent and the nursing staff were converted to patient rooms.

The Nurses' Training Schools

Although nursing must certainly have played an important role in the care of patients during the early years of Miners' Hospital No. 2, none of the biennial reports prior to 1910 mention the nursing staff. The 1910 biennial report of the State Board of Control of West Virginia does provide a glimpse of who provided nursing care at the hospital and explains why the administration believed a training school must be established.[24] From the report it can be surmised that prior to 1910 the nursing staff was comprised of graduate nurses and students from regional training schools.[25] Although it was the largest of the three hospitals, Miners' Hospital No. 1 continued to use graduate nurses exclusively until it established its training school in 1914.[26] The apparent catalyst for the establishment of the McKendree training school was efficiency. By having its own nursing students the hospital did not have to rely on other institutions to supply graduate nurses, and their own students would be reliable and readily available at any time of the day or night. Miners' Hospital No. 3 opened its training school in 1903 for the same reason, to avoid labor problems associated with graduate nurses.[27]

THE NURSING WORKFORCE AND STAFFING ISSUES
AT MCKENDREE HOSPITAL NO. 2

On the basis of the traumatic injuries incurred by the miners and other laborers of the region, nursing at McKendree Hospital No. 2 had to have been, at the very least, rigorous and not unlike nursing in the other miners' hospitals. Accident victims came by train night and day. The patient records and hospital registers suggest that many patients were simply cleaned, examined, treated, and released. However, many more were admitted, which meant limbs had to be amputated, bones set, wounds sewn, and burns treated. A large number of surgical and orthopedic cases were admitted, and care of these patients with major trauma required prolonged intensive postoperative nursing care. In record after record, explosions and cave-ins or slate slides are mentioned. These mishaps resulted in crushed limbs, skulls, and backs. At the time, there were surgical methods to repair and stabilize skull fractures and spines; however, few patients with these injuries survived. Those with massive crushing of the lower limbs, particularly the femur, had a poor chance of survival. Many poor souls were simply cleaned and comforted during their final hours.

To put the number of injuries requiring surgical intervention into perspective, an examination of the records for McKendree Hospital No. 2 reveals that in 1910, 557 surgeries were performed: by 1916 the number rose to 620 per year. It appears from the records that 45% of all patients admitted to McKendree during these 6 years required some form of surgical intervention. Staffing the wards of these hospitals with nurses must have been an incredible challenge for the Superintendent of Nurses and the hospital administrators despite the fact that nursing students worked 12-hour shifts from 8:00 until 8:00.

The 1910 biennial report for Miners' Hospital No. 2 lists the daily average number of patients as twenty-nine. The maximum number of patients in one day could be as high as forty. As the years went on, the census continued to increase in all of the hospitals. However, the number of nurses available to care for the patients does not appear to have kept pace with the increased numbers of patients. By 1912 a head nurse was employed at McKendree Hospital No. 2, and the number of students had increased to six. At least one nurse was required to be in the operating room during surgeries. The daily average of patients that year increased to thirty-three, and the daily maximum increased to forty-six. The biennial report for 1916 reveals little improvement in the nurse-to-patient ratio. The hospital's capacity increased and, as was mentioned earlier, was in the process of being increased again with the addition of the nurses' home and the resultant space released for patient beds. The number of nurses listed for 1916 was nine, in addition to the Superintendent of Nurses. While the number of nurses may at first appear to be reasonable, it must be kept in mind that all of the nurses would not be working each shift but were divided between the two shifts. The required nursing staff in the operating room further reduced the number of students available to work on the hospital wards. The work and care on the wards was generally accomplished by one or two registered nurses supervising the students, who performed most of the care.[28]

MORTALITY RATES

Mortality rates were a constant concern for the administrators of the hospitals, and detailed death records were maintained. In 1902 the death rate at Miners' Hospital No. 2 was 14%, and the rate increased as the census rose. The highest recorded death rate occurred in 1906 when McKendree saw an appalling 20.5% death rate. It should be noted that many of the deaths occurred 1-2 hours after admission because of the victims' extensive trauma. In 1910, the year the training school at McKendree opened, the mortality rate was still 14%. However, after the opening of the training school the death rates declined dramatically despite the continual increase in patient numbers. By 1913 the mortality rate had dropped to 3%, and 1915 saw a death rate of 5%.

Miners' Hospital No. 1 reported mortality rates ranging from 10% to over 14%, in the years prior to the establishment of its training school. Miners' Hospital No. 3 had the lowest mortality rates between the years 1902 and 1910, with the rate ranging between 3.5 and 5.5%. Miners' Hospital No. 3 was also the first to establish a nurses' training school, seeking a more reliable nursing staff.

There is no direct evidence to suggest that there was a major change in the hospitals' administrators, surgical techniques, or statistical methods that could account for the significant lowering of mortality rates during the years recorded above. However, one factor shared by all three hospitals was the establishment of the training schools. The establishment of the training schools provided an organized system of nursing care in which to train the students. A reliable work force of nursing students could also have lead to overall improved patient care, resulting in decreased mortality.

TRAUMA CARE IN THE MINERS' HOSPITALS

The patient records and hospital registers from 1909 and 1916 truly reveal what life as a McKendree nurse must have been like. As mentioned earlier, at the time, there were surgical methods to repair and stabilize skull fractures.[29,30] However, spinal injuries and paralysis proved to be more daunting.[31,32]

Postoperative infections were always a threat to the survival of surgical cases. Many patients survived the extensive surgeries but later developed and succumbed to infections. Burns and their resultant secondary infections were also a challenge and often did not have a positive prognosis or outcome.

164   John C. Kirchgessner

Infections were treated with compounds containing mercury, phenol, alcohol, and arsenic. Mercury compounds were used for their disinfectant properties and were considered to be one of the most powerful germicides of the time. However, mercury was not without side effects, and warnings were abundant in references regarding its use. Arsenic was believed to be particularly helpful in skin infections and was frequently used.[33]

THE CARE OF MEDICAL CASES

Although the majority of cases seen at the miners' hospitals were surgical in nature, there were medical problems dealt with as well. Conjunctivitis, eczema, gastritis, orchitis, and nephritis are but a few of the medical diagnoses listed in McKendree's second biennial report of 1912. While the hospitals were originally established for acute care and people with infectious diseases were not intentionally admitted, patients were often diagnosed with infectious diseases after admission and required care. Malaria, tuberculosis, and typhoid were some of the infectious diseases that had to be managed. Whether all of these cases were diagnosed after admission or patients were knowingly admitted with these diseases is not clear. It was not unusual for similar hospitals of this era to loosely abide by their infectious disease regulations. It is important to keep in mind that the miners' hospitals were the only healthcare facilities in these relatively remote regions. When outbreaks of infectious diseases occurred, such as the three mentioned above, the hospitals and their administrators may have had little choice but to respond in order to keep the greater community as healthy as possible.

Women and children were also admitted to the miners' hospitals. As the years went on, the hospital's biennial reports' statistics indicate an increase in the number of women and children receiving care. As a result of this change in patient population, nurses not only were required to have knowledge in surgical and medical nursing, they also needed to know pediatrics and womens' health. During the early years of McKendree's training school is not clear where the nursing students received their formal training in these specialties, if indeed they did receive any. The physicians' lectures were possibly one source of this knowledge. In later years, however, the nursing students were sent to Cincinnati for education and training in pediatrics and women's health.[34]

Conclusion

The coal industry brought many hardships and changes to the state of West Virginia. Possibly the greatest change was in the status of the people. Once self-supporting farmers and mountaineers, the West Virginians of the early 20th century became dependent employees, often with few benefits to show for their years of literally "back- breaking" work. Prior to the establishment of the state's miners' hospitals, healthcare was minimal, partly because of the remoteness of the coal fields and partly because of the lack of interest by physicians in establishing practices in such regions. The major industries, too, showed little interest in providing anything other than minimal healthcare for their employees and their families. The opening of the miners' hospitals provided hope for healthcare of the coal miners and their families. Nursing had a direct impact on the improvement of patient care in the hospitals. Although the hospitals had many limitations that prohibited their ability to provide optimal care and it is not exactly clear what impact the hospitals had on the region's healthcare, they did meet a need and organize healthcare in an industrial region that had never had such care. It was a never-ending cycle of admitting, stabilizing, and comforting people under conditions that were not always ideal.

JOHN C. KIRCHGESSNER, MSN, RN, PNP
School of Nursing
McLeod Hall
University of Virginia
Charlotesville, VA 22903

Notes

1. C. A. Frazier, *Miners and Medicine: West Virginia Memories* (Norman, Okla.: University of Oklahoma Press, 1992), 43. "The state had the unenviable reputation of being the mining state least concerned about the safety and welfare of its workers. One West Virginia governor allegedly remarked that it was entirely natural that miners should be injured and killed in the course of their labors. The coal companies literally got away with murder well into the twentieth century."

2. M. Bragg, *Window to the Past, Part III: McKendree Miners' Hospital* (Glen Jean, W.V.: GEM Publications, n.d.), 1.

3. Frazier, *Miners and Medicine*, 38. "In 1915, West Virginia amended its child-labor law to make it illegal for children under . . . sixteen to work in mines."

4. *Acts of the Legislature of West Virginia*, 1907, Charleston, W.Va., State Archives, p. 330.

5. Frazier, *Miners and Medicine*, 34.

6. Ibid., 58. "Thus, before the railroads made their way into the mountains of Appalachia, hardy mountain folk had to rely entirely on themselves in sickness as well as in health. Beyond the town boundaries there were no physicians, no hospitals, no pharmacies."

7. Ibid., 88. "The arrival of the first coal company doctors was a medical breakthrough for the people of Appalachia; however, for many years those doctors manned a lonely bastion, and both they and their seriously ill or injured patients soon realized more was needed. The nearest hospital was still a long, rough wagon ride or an infrequent train trip away. The end result of a trip to the hospital was too often to arrive dead on arrival."

8. Bragg, *Window to the Past,* 1. "Local doctors saw their quiet family practices turn into a nightmare as they were suddenly faced with a growing tide of men with arms, legs, and even skulls, crushed by rock falls."

9. *Acts of the Legislature of West Virginia,* 1899, Charleston, W.Va., State Archives, p. 176.

10. Ibid., 178.

11. *Biennial Report of Miners' Hospital No. 2,* 1904, Charleston, W.Va., State Archives, p. 11.

[A] glance at the list of occupations of patients admitted shows that while, naturally, the miners predominate largely there is a fair representation of the other callings of a district necessarily limited in interests. As nearly as possible in all cases a literal representation of the law governing the admission of patients into these hospitals has been observed. Medical cases have not been admitted as free patients into this hospital and in a number of instances have been refused as pay cases on account of lack of or improper accommodations. In several instances acute surgical cases in women, eligible under the law, have been refused on account of lack of accommodations.

12. *Acts of the Legislature of West Virginia,* 1903, Charleston, W.Va., State Archives, p. 163.

13. West Virginia, State Archives, *Acts of the Legislature* (1899), 176.

14. Ibid., 177.

15. Ibid., 179.

16. Ibid., 176.

17. McKendree, Fayette Co., *Report of Miners 'Hospital No. 2,* 1902, Charleston, W.Va., State Archives, p. 5. "The locality is practically isolated, with no society, school, or church facilities for its of officials. . . ." In addition, the Board of Directors had concerns about the hospital's isolation and the need for larger facilities should patient acuity demand it. "Also, no fast trains stop at McKendree, and should a patient be sent there upon a local train, a distance of fifty to seventy-five miles, he would have lost instead of gained anything in the way of time consumed en routes. . . ."

18. Bragg, *Window to the Past,* 2. "The community of McKendree was on the main line of the C&O Railway . . . When completed, Miners' Hospital No. 2 sat on a tract of land . . . one-fourth mile east of the McKendree station. The tract of land was on the side of the mountain, fifty feet above and one hundred feet back, from the railroad tracks." The fact that the hospital was a quarter of a mile from the local depot and fifty feet up a mountainside is significant in how patients were transported from the depot to the hospital. In later years, transportation of newly arrived patients would be a concern as the census increased at Miners' Hospital No. 2.

19. *Miners' Hospital No. 2,* 1902, W. Va., State Archives, p. 5.

20. *Biennial Report West Virginia Miners' Hospital No. 3,* 1902, Charleston, W.Va., State Archives, p. 2.

21. *Biennial Report West Virginia Miners' Hospital No. 1,* 1904, W. Va., State Archives, p. 4.

22. *Miners' Hospital No. 3,* 15.

23. *Fourth Biennial of the State Board of Control of West Virginia for the Period 1 July 1914 to 30 June 1916,* W. Va., State Archives, p. 222.

[A] contract is let and work begun on the building of a nurses' home which when complete will be a modern brick building furnishing ample room for twenty nurses . . . We will then be able to convert that part of the hospital . . . for the accommodation of patients, thus giving us about ten private rooms.

24. *First Biennial Report of the State Board of Control of West Virginia for the Biennial Period Ending September 30, 1910,* Charleston, W.Va., State Archives, p.131. "In order that we might have more efficient help, that we would be independent of other Training Schools and graduate nurses, we deemed it necessary to establish a training school, which was done March 1, 1910 . . ."

25. *Second Biennial Report of the State Board of Control of West Virginia for the Biennial Period Ending September 30, 1912,* W. Va., State Archives, p. 180. "We are proud of the feet that we are able to get better service and more conscientious work than when we employed graduates."

26. *Fourth Biennial Report of the Board of Control of West Virginia, July 1, 1914 to June 30, 1916,* Charleston, W.Va., State Archives, p. 202.

27. *Second Biennial Report of the Board of Directors, Superintendent, Secretary and Treasurer of Miners' Hospital No. 3,* 1904, Charleston, W.Va., State Archives, p. 21.

28. Frazier, *Miners and Medicine,* 99. "You could hear the ambulances rolling in with mining emergency cases and regardless of who you were working for, doctors would step out into the hall and call out, 'A little help here!' . . . And all available nurses would run to help."

29. Bragg, *Window to the Past,* 14. The following excerpt from a 1909 patient record explains how a young man's fractured skull was surgically repaired. "Fracture of skull was first operated upon and fractured bone removed. Gauze drainage was put in and the wound closed."

30. Ibid., 14. Another entry in the 1909 patient record reveals a thirty year old man was admitted with the diagnosis of fracture of the skull and compound fractures of the frontal bone and laceration of brain tissues and ". . . taken to the dressing room where chloroform was administered and his wound dressed . . . several pieces of bone being removed from the brain substance. Died at 7:20 o'clock a.m."

31. Ibid., 18. A patient record from 1909 of a forty year old man who received a fractured spine in a slate fall describes his four months at McKendree. "Patient has complete paralysis of left leg. Also of right leg from lower third of thigh. Retention of urine and feces. Catheterized every 8 hours. 10/30: Condition not much improved. Trophic sores on back. 11/29: No improvement in patient's condition. Bad sores developing rapidly. 1/3: Shows no improvement. 1/24: 8 a.m. Died."

32. *Third Biennial Report of the State Board of Control of West Virginia for the Period October 1, 1912 to June 30, 1914*, W. Va., State Archives, p. 258. Dr. Wheeler, hospital superintendent for McKendree Hospital No. 2, specifically addressed spinal trauma in his report for 1914, noting that there had been fourteen deaths that years due to broken backs, ". . . a condition for which at the present time surgery does not offer much in the way of cure." Dr. Wheeler's report further reveals that few patients with severe head injury, spinal trauma, and the resulting paralysis survived.

33. C. Weeks-Shaw, *A Text-Book of Nursing* (New York: D. Appleton and Company, 1903), 104, 143, 145.

34. W. E. Cox, *National Park Service, New River Gorge NR Archives, Interview 33—Nursing*, 1981, 33.17, New River Gorge NR Cultural Resources Library, Glen Jean, W. Va.

A Hard Day's Work
Institutional Nursing in the Post-World War II Era

Victoria T. Grando

The University of Missouri-Columbia
Sinclair School of Nursing

At the end of World War II the hospital industry in the United States was booming, driven largely by postwar prosperity and the dramatic rise in private health insurance plans.[1] As money became increasingly available for health care, hospitals were becoming centers of high technology, where more and more people went for surgery and acute care.[2] Numerous factors precipitated this new demand for services including an increase in the elderly population, a high postwar birth rate, and numerous disabled veterans needing services.[3] At the same time, institutional nursing faced numerous challenges. Low salaries, meager benefits, and long hours continued to plague hospital nursing as they had done since nurses began working for hospitals as general duty nurses in the mid-1930s.[4] However, after the sacrifices of World War II (WWII) staff nurses were increasingly restless with their working conditions and wanted improvements.[5] Here I describe and analyze post-WWII hospital nurses' working conditions, nurses' reactions to their working conditions, and the reasons why many continued to work in institutional nursing in spite of the numerous drawbacks. These nursing events are viewed within the larger frame of women's lives and work patterns in the 1940s and 1950s.

American Women in the Postwar Years

The postwar era was a time when the country spent its energies and resources on economic growth and the stabilization of family life.[6] The mood of the country was one of consensus, conservatism, and family centeredness.[7] Women took part in advancing the American dream by assuring social stability through

Nursing History Review 8 (2000): 169-184. A publication of the American Association for the History of Nursing. Copyright © 2000 Springer Publishing Company.

their role at home, commitment to their families, and responsibility for their children's and husbands' welfare.[8] However, historians have argued that this domestic role, which Betty Friedan coined the "feminine mystique," did not provide a base from which women could assert themselves, engage in social reform, or build strong female bonds.[9] Sara Evans pointed out, "There was no strong sense of public or civic life where women could put into practice the values of domesticity, nor were those values easily expressed in communal terms."[10] Rather, it was through accommodation and adaptation that women made their relationships and marriages work.[11]

The central role "family" played in society had a great impact on women's lives because women of the era were defined primarily by their roles of wife and mother. Indeed, as William H. Chafe and others maintain, any stress at home or discontent with the roles of wife and mother was labeled pathological.[12] Both women and men believed that women should be fulfilled with their families at home. Many women preferred homemaking to careers in the labor market because they felt it offered them independence and autonomy. This was also true for many Black women who saw the role of the wife, devoting all her energies to homemaking, as a goal for which to strive. Only a small minority of well-educated middle-class White women were discontent with the narrowness of their gender-defined roles.[13]

Institutional Nursing

Within this context, hospital nursing took shape after WWII. The wages of hospital nurses in the postwar period were lower than those of many other workers, a fact underscored by the U.S. Department of Labor report, *The Economic Status of Registered Professional Nurses, 1946-47.* It stressed the inadequacy of nurses' salaries with the following: "there are occupations in this country requiring much less training that provide hourly pay equal to or above that of most nurses."[14]

Comparing the wages of hospital nurses with other women workers of this era reveals the extent of the problem. According to the 1950 Census reports the median yearly salaries in 1949 for most female professionals were higher than those for nurses. Nurses' median yearly salaries were $2,127.00. This was lower than the salaries of female teachers, $2,394.00; female social workers, $2,497.00; and female physicians, $3,475.00. The wages of hospital nurses faired no better when compared to nonprofessional groups. Female stenographers, typists, and secretaries were averaging a slightly higher annual salary than nurses, $2,138.00.

In addition, the average hourly wage for institutional nurses in 1946 was $0.87, while the average hourly wage for bookkeepers was $1.15, women assemblers in the machinery industry (requiring little special training) earned $1.00 per hour, and women garment workers in the suit and coat industry averaged $1.47.[15]

Frustration Over Wages

Many, in and out of nursing, believed that nurses' meager wages stemmed from hospital administrators' practice of balancing hospital budgets by keeping salaries low.[16] In 1946, Emily Hicks wrote a series of three articles on nurses' labor status in *The Trained Nurse and Hospital Review*. She argued that hospitals historically kept nursing labor costs at a minimum. This began with their early reliance on free student labor and continued as hospitals started employing graduate nurses. She held that hospital management persisted in the belief that nursing costs must continue to be "rock bottom" because hospitals saw themselves as charitable institutions. This philosophy led hospital administrators to keep nurses' salaries down during WWII and in the immediate postwar era. They did this, Hicks maintained, in spite of the fact that during this period, hospitals had higher operating budgets resulting from rising room rates while retaining low personnel costs.[17] Similarly, Janet M. Giester objected to hospitals' claiming that they could not afford higher salaries while they were able to erect large additions and purchase new equipment.[18]

Moreover as Norman Metzger and Dennis Pointer argue in their book on hospital labor-management relations, hospitals had a "bimodal mix" or "hourglass" personnel structure until the early 1960s. This meant that employees received either a relatively high-level or a relatively low-level rate of pay with few in the middle range. They held that because most hospital employees were women, a group that have been historically underpaid, this further depressed hospital salaries, and they believed that the lack of unionization on the part of hospital employees was an important reason why wages were kept low.[19]

The fact that nurses' salaries were lower than those of many other workers in the nation troubled nurses.[20] Nurses' discontent over their wages was echoed at the Thirty-Fifth American Nurses' Association (ANA) Convention in 1946 with a vote for minimal adequate salaries and by numerous staff nurses' letters to nursing journals.[21] One nurse expressed the feelings of many nurses at the end of WWII in a letter to the editors of *American Journal of Nursing*. She wrote the following:

Nurses like nursing—they are proud of their responsibility, their ability to aid the sick, but they are realistic as well as idealistic. Domestic help, beauty operators, and waitresses receive, in most instances, a higher salary than hospital staff nurses . . . It isn't difficult to discover the reason for inadequate hospital personnel.[22]

The frustration over salaries led some to quit hospital nursing.[23] In an editorial in *R.N.*, Alice Clarke claimed that nurses were revolting over their dissatisfaction with economic conditions that had been mounting for years. She stated the following:

For years, there has been an almost silent revolutionary movement among nurses . . . Noiselessly, nurses have crept out of nursing not making too much ado. These mute escapists have brought about the present crisis (nursing shortage).[24]

Married nurses were especially dissatisfied with their low wages and gave that as a reason for not working. They claimed that hospital wages did not cover the expenses incurred when working.[25] A married nurse quoted in the 1947 government report, *The Economic Status of Registered Professional Nurses, 1946-1947*, stated the following:

For the average married nurse with children, the hourly rate of 8 1/2 cents is insufficient. Day nurseries require a minimum of $14 per child for 5 days a week. . . . it really does not pay me to go to work as much as I would sincerely like to help out in the nursing shortage.[26]

Burdens of Staff Nursing

Although salaries were an important issue, institutional nurses also viewed poor working conditions as a critical issue.[27] Work schedules were especially troublesome, a fact that limited nurses' social life.[28] In the late 1940s, nurses worked long hours. The average number of hours worked was 48 hours a week, while over 30% of them worked more than 50 hours. A few, often those working night shifts, actually worked 60 and 72 hours per week.[29] The *American Journal of Nursing* reported that delegates to the 1946 ANA biennial convention were more concerned with limiting the number of hours worked than with maximizing salaries. According to the article "they (nurses) wanted freedom *to live* (italic in original) as well as to work."[30] The disenchantment of one general staff nurse, Beverly White, conveys some of the frustration felt by nurses about their working conditions. She wrote the following in an *American Journal of Nursing* article responding to public criticism of nursing:

> My work load is heavy; I don't have time to be gentle and indulgent! My awful hours do not permit me to live a decent life of my own! . . . The work is so monotonous, so routinized, there is nothing creative about it, nothing to keep my interest renewed![31]

Nurses' work schedules compared unfavorably with the national trend for other workers. During the mid-1940s other women workers had shorter, more regular hours than nurses. Female production workers in manufacturing averaged only slightly under 40 hours a week, and most women in office work averaged 40 hours week.[32] Moreover, in some cases, improvements that nurses were seeking did not even meet the minimum standards set by the government. In 1945, fourteen state nurses' associations were attempting to upgrade personnel practices by asking for a 48-hour week.[33] This was still far above the 40-hour work week set in 1933 by the National Recovery Administration.[34]

Work schedules were also a point of dissatisfaction. One scheduling pattern, split shifts, was disliked by many staff nurses. Split shifts meant that a nurse might work 8 or 9 hours a day, but these hours were broken up by 3-4 hours off in the middle of a 12-hour shift. Nurses who worked them complained that time off in the middle of a shift was most often wasted and of little benefit. They preferred to work straight shifts with no interruptions.[35]

Little advance notice of days off also frustrated nurses. Many worked 6 days a week with short notice of regularly scheduled hours or days off.[36] In 1947, 19% of institutional nurses' hours were posted either the same day or 1 day in advance of days off, while 49% of institutional nurses' hours were scheduled from 1 week to 10 days in advance of days off.[37]

Other practices that affected work schedules were emergency call and overtime work. A quarter of institutional nurses were "on call." The majority of them worked from 1 to 20 extra hours a month. The study *The Economic Status of Registered Professional Nurses, 1946–1947*, showed that 63.5% of institutional nurses worked overtime. Furthermore, 38% of these received no pay or time off for overtime work and 3% received time and a half.[38]

The demoralization from low pay and long hours was exacerbated by heavy work loads.[39] Nurses believed that their patient work loads were excessive and questioned if these heavy workloads compromised patient safety.[40] Geister reported that many nurses were more dissatisfied in 1948 than during the depression because of the increase in the number of patients they had to care for. This resulted, she maintained, because hospitals' census were high and nurses' case loads were 3-4 times heavier. At the same time, hospitals were putting the "new money" (i.e., insurance money) into equipment and buildings rather than into increasing nurses' pay or employing a sufficient number of nurses.[41]

One group that was especially adamant about their displeasure with hospital nursing was returning nurse veterans of WWII.[42] They hoped that low salaries and poor working conditions would improve at the end of the war, but many found conditions unchanged. As a result, some opted for new jobs in and out of nursing.[43] Bertha Mears, a frustrated nursing superintendent trying to attract returning veterans to her hospital, echoed the sentiment of returning military nurses with the following:

> No, they [nurses on terminal military leave] were not interested in coming back. They did not know just what they were going to do, but they did know that they were never going to work in a hospital again. They had talked it over while overseas, and nearly everyone felt the same way . . . Yes, hospital work was far more interesting, and they really missed it terribly. But—never again! There was more to life than just working oneself to death.[44]

The extent of nurse veterans' frustration was captured in a survey done by the ANA of returning army nurses. Of the 31,000 who responded to the questionnaire, 69% said that they planned to return to nursing, but only 16% were planning to return to their prewar position.[45]

The hierarchical structure in hospitals also irritated some staff nurses. Hospitals operated on an authoritarian system with nursing services often caught between hospital bureaucracy and the medical staff. Although physicians were not part of the formal hospital structure, they depended on nurses to obey their every order.[46] Consequently, nurses were expected to be obedient and unquestioning and were often fired for being outspoken.[47] Moreover, their role was seen by some as simply carrying out doctors' orders and merely being timesavers for physicians.[48] Dorothy Wheeler, a Director of Nursing, believed that the nursing shortage resulted from nurses' dissatisfaction with hospital hierarchy and said the following:

> The nurses want to feel that they have a share in what hospitals are accomplishing and are not just a small segment which takes orders. They want a part in matters of policy.[49]

An editorial in *New York Medicine* expressing surprise at her views illustrates a physician's perspective of the situation:

If a nurse looks upon herself as primarily a professional person, . . . ,under the necessary and natural supervision of physicians, it is hard to understand what matters of policy she will be especially concerned with.[50]

Societal Pressures Influence Nursing Manpower

As the Brown Report concluded, it was amazing that women continued to work in nursing or choose it as a career given the working conditions in the postwar era.[51] Considering that there were increasing numbers of jobs available for women with better hours, pay, and working conditions, one is led to wonder: Why did many nurses continue to work in hospitals when hours were long, benefits were few, and salaries were so bad?[52] One RN in 1948 expressed this very sentiment in a letter to the editor of *R.N.* with the following observation,

> For the past several years I have read innumerable letters to the *R.N.* magazine from registered nurses complaining bitterly against their profession. Long hours, little remuneration, bullying, belittling experiences and many other vituperative remarks—complaining without end. It is a wonder to me these misguided people remain in the profession.[53]

To understand why nurses stayed, it is important to examine the forces shaping women's work before, during, and after the postwar period as well as forces within the healthcare delivery system.

Propaganda during World War II stressed the importance and value of women not only as wives and mothers but also as workers. The necessity of increased labor power during the war and the shortage of men to fill the positions made it possible for many women to transcend traditional gender roles and work outside the home in large numbers. It became patriotic for women to leave their homes and work. Between 1940 and 1945, over 6 million women, both single and married, entered the labor force. Female workers made gains in all fields of employment, including jobs that had previously been exclusively held by males, such as those in heavy industry. In fact, the only work role for women that did not increase during the war was domestic service.[54]

Although the war had greatly disrupted established roles for American women, its end saw little change in social expectations for them. After World War II the barriers against women reappeared; women doing men's work and getting paid higher wages had been acceptable for the duration of the war only. Long-held gender ideology, as well as the uncertainties caused by both the cold war and the onset of the nuclear age, prevented the breakdown in gender-defined roles from having a lasting effect. Popular literature at the end of the war admonished women to put the needs of the returning men above their own, to forsake the independence and assertiveness they developed during World War II, and to cultivate feminine qualities. As the men returned from the war fronts women were pushed out of their new jobs, and there was a renewed belief in the primacy of women's domestic role within the family.[55] Even the fact that large numbers of women left the confines of private life during the war to enter the job market did not alter this. As Chafe summarized, "Women's sphere had been expanded, yet traditional attitudes toward woman's place remained largely unchanged."[56]

In spite of the belief that mothers should stay home and tend their families, women could legitimately work as long as they did not have very young children and worked to augment their family's income. Moreover, as Chafe and others have argued, the war did little to change women's work force participation. Rather, economic pressures and the realization that women's paid work outside the home was important in raising the family's standard of living were the driving forces that changed women's work patterns in the 1950s. This shift in women's work patterns persisted into the 1960s and included the following changes: (1) the beginning of a societal acceptance of women working outside the home and a substantial increase in the number of women working; (2) the continued segregation of women in low-paying jobs with few opportunities for advancement, such as clerical and service jobs; (3) the increased opportunities for women in the female semiprofessions; (4) the declining numbers of young women available to work and rising numbers of older women in the work force, and (5) continued emphasis on part-time work with growing numbers of women choosing full-time work.[57]

Some aspects of the changing women's job market influenced the nursing labor supply. In particular, the increased competition for women workers hurt nursing. As a result of it, nursing found itself vying for new recruits as young women had new job options.[58] In fact, there was a sharp decline in nursing school enrollments, coupled with an increase in nursing school dropouts after the war.[59] Indeed, 1947 was a dismal year for nursing schools. Nursing school enrollments dropped from 128,828 in 1946 to 106,900 in 1947, a decline of 17%. Enrollments continued to decline until 1950.[60] This drop in nursing school enrollments was unexpected since enrollments had been on a steady rise before and during the war.[61] At the same time, however, some of the changes had a positive effect on nursing's manpower. In particular, the increases in older women and mothers working swelled the nursing ranks. In fact, ANA held that much of the growth in nurses' ranks in the late 1950s and early 1960s was due to inactive nurses returning to work and not to new recruits.[62]

Why Nurses Stayed on the Job

Within this larger backdrop of growing women's work opportunities and changing work patterns, nursing continued to hold an attraction for many women. This occurred for reasons both within society and within the healthcare delivery system. For one thing, nursing embodied the feminine roles of caring and nurturing during this era that stressed a women's domestic role and putting others first. Eugenia Kaledin argues that women of the postwar period found strength in achievements within their domestic confines and did not believe that they had to compete in male arenas. Furthermore, she holds that women tried to extend their values of caring and nurturing into other aspects of their lives.[63] Not surprisingly, many women sincerely enjoyed nursing or believed that the satisfaction of nursing others was more important than the monetary rewards of nursing.[64] In a letter to the editor of *American Journal of Nursing* a nurse expresses that sentiment in the following:

> Salary raises and shorter hours are nice, but I would dislike feeling that money is the only return for a few hours longer on duty to see a patient get well. . . . I feel repaid in my efforts when I see them improved and grateful.[65]

Moreover, many nurses felt that nursing was important women's work that afforded them status within their communities. They saw nursing as essential and believed that it played a vital role in a patient's recovery. As one nurse, quoted in the *American Journal of Nursing*, put it:

> There *may* [italics in the original] be some more interesting occupation than nursing. . . . but I do not know what it could be. The suspense of watching a patient's physical and psychological reaction to good care is dramatic. Until you see a patient whom you expected to die walk out of the hospital, you don't know what durable satisfactions are.[66]

Some nurses also felt that it prepared them to be better mothers.[67]

Another societal force included the strong expectation within American culture that nurses had the duty to minister to the sick. Indeed, nurses were being pressured by the media to provide nursing care after World War II.[68]

Several articles appeared in the lay press expressing concern about the nursing shortages.[69] One article, "What Happens When Trained Nurses Won't Nurse the Sick?" by Gretta Palmer, was especially negative about nurses' alleged unwillingness to work under prevailing conditions in hospitals.[70] It prompted much discussion within the nursing community.[71] As a result, some nurses persevered in their jobs because they believed the nation needed them.[72] Society's drastic need for registered nurses also influenced nurses by effectively legitimizing working in an era that expected women to stay home.[73] Thus it provided married nurses with an acceptable reason to work for pay.[74]

There were also forces operating within the healthcare delivery system that were effective in keeping nurses on the job, especially the organizational structure of nursing schools and hospitals. Schools of nursing had a long history of authoritarianism and expecting self-sacrifice from nursing students. Indeed, from the beginning of their nursing careers student nurses were indoctrinated in unquestioning obedience.[75] This was intensified as they became staff nurses. Hospital's organizational hierarchy fostered subservience, obedience, and a sense of duty on the part of nurses.[76] This led to nurses accepting the status quo in hospitals and made it more likely that they would remain on the job.[77] Shirley Titus, a California nurse who worked diligently for nurses' economic security, argued this point in 1952 in an article in the *American Journal of Nursing*:

> Because the nurse spends most of her waking hours in an environment which is dominated by hospital management and doctors, she has remained far more docile, if not actually subservient, than perhaps any other American worker. Hospital management and organized medicine have not only shaped in part the world of nursing but they have also conditioned the thinking of nurses. And the nurse has accepted the thinking of these two groups—especially in regard to her status, her function, and her social and economic welfare—with amazingly little demur or question."[78]

Conclusions

The interaction of numerous societal forces in the post-World War II era played a crucial part in shaping nurses' decisions about work. Although more women worked outside the home, job options were limited to traditional women's work, and barriers to well-paying jobs remained. Women's sphere of influence remained in the home, and their role as caregiver was emphasized. At the same time, there was a grave shortage of nurses caused by changes within the healthcare system that created increased need, as many nurses at the end of the war chose to remain home. This led the American press to question why nurses stopped working, with some blaming nurses for not wanting to nurse the sick. In addition, the widespread low salaries, the poor working conditions, and an authoritarian structure in hospitals gave nurses few employment choices.

Nurses for the most part accepted the prevailing views of both the larger culture and the hospital culture. As a result, they, just like other women of the era, did what was expected them. They put family first, worked to help out their family, and enjoyed doing women's work in both their private and public lives. Thus women chose nursing because it was viewed as acceptable, fulfilling work for women that enhanced their role as mother. Furthermore, many nurses felt obliged to provide nursing care at a time when nurses were so badly needed. Consequently, many of them continued to work in hospitals even though they were overworked and poorly paid.

At the same time, however, some nurses began organizing through the American Nurses Association's Economic Security Program as a way to change their working conditions and ensure quality nursing care. This was an important step for nurses because they were becoming proactive in an era that did not encourage women to take up social causes. Also, they began the long road toward improving working conditions and wages by setting employment standards and establishing collective bargaining.[79] Although the Economic Security Program had a slow beginning, nurses for the first time at all levels were articulating their economic wants as a group and working collectively to meet them.[80]

VICTORIA I. GRANDO, RN, PHD
Sinclair School of Nursing
The University of Missouri-Columbia
Columbia, MO, 65211

Notes

1. Paul Starr, *The Social Transformation of American Medicine* (New York: Basic Books, 1982), 335.
2. Rosemary Stevens, *In Sickness and in Wealth: American Hospitals in the Twentieth Century* (New York: Basic Books, 1989), 227–228.
3. U.S. Department of Labor, Bureau of Labor Statistics, *The Economic Status of Registered Professional Nurses*, BLS bulletin 931 (Washington, D.C.: U.S.

Government Printing Office, 1947), 4; Aryness J. Wickens, "A Social and Economic Poll of Nurses," *The American Journal of Nursing* 46 (November 1946): 755 (hereafter cited as AJN).

4. Esther L. Brown, *Nursing for the Future: A Report Prepared for the National Nursing Council* (New York: Russell Sage Foundation, 1948), 45–47; U.S. Department of Labor, *Economic Status*, 4; Susan M. Reverby, *Ordered to Care: The Dilemma of American Nursing* (Cambridge, U.K.: Cambridge University Press, 1987), 191–95.

5. "The ANA Economic Security Program," AJN 47 (February 1947): 70; Florence Brannigan, "Why Army Nurses Leave Nursing," AJN 46 (January 1946): 56. Ruth E. Sutter, "Letters-Pro and Con: Salaries," AJN 46 (May 1946): 328; Civilian Nurse, "Letters-Pro and Con: Salaries," AJN 46 (May 1946): 328; Marley Jo Bready, "Letters-Pro and Con: The Reason?" AJN 46 (October 1946): 706; R.N., "Letters-Pro and Con: Collective Bargaining," AJN 46 (October 1946): 706.

6. Marty Jezer, *The Dark Ages: Life in the United States, 1945–1965* (Boston: South End Press, 1982), 117–33; William L. O'Neill, *American High: The Years of Confidence, 1945–1960* (New York: Free Press, 1986), 33–44.

7. Jezer, *The Dark Ages*, 118–9; O'Neill, *American High*, 6–7.

8. O'Neill, *American High*, 7, 40–41; Susan M. Hartmann, *American Women in the 1940s: The Home Front and Beyond* (Boston: Twayne Publishing, 1982), 16; Elaine T. May, *Homeward Bound: American Families in the Cold War* (New York: Basic Books, 1988), 28–29; Sara M. Evans, *Born to Liberty: A History of Women in America* (New York: The Free Press, 1989), 244–47.

9. Feminine mystique was the term coined by Betty Friedan in her best-selling book about the dilemma of women's lifestyle from the late 1940s through the early 1960s. Betty Friedan, *The Feminine Mystique* (New York: W.W. Norton & Company, 1983); Evans, *Born to Liberty*, 255; Rochelle Gatlin, *American Women Since 1945* (Jackson, Miss.: University Press of Mississippi, 1987), 12.

10. Evans, *Born to Liberty*, 255.

11. May, *Homeward Bound*, 183

12. William H. Chafe, *The Paradox of Change: American Women in the 20th Century* (New York: Oxford University Press, 1991), 176–86; Hartmann, *Home Front*, 213; May, *Homeward Bound*, 187, Gatlin, *American Women*, 16.

13. Chafe, *The Paradox of Change*, 175–93; Hartmann, *Home Front*, 213; May, *Homeward Bound*, 28–29; Gatlin, *American Women*, 17.

14. U.S. Department of Labor, *Economic Status*, 51.

15. U.S. Bureau of the Census, Characteristics of the Population, *U.S. Census of Population: 1950*, pt. 1 (Washington, D.C.: U.S. Government Printing Office, 1953) II: 281–282; U.S. Department of Labor, *Economic Status*, 12, 51; U.S. Department of Labor, Women's Bureau, *Handbook of Facts on Women Workers*, bulletin no. 225 (Washington, D.C.: U.S. Government Printing Office, 1948), 27. One needs to be careful when examining nurses wage data; often one figure is reported for all nurses in administration, education, public health, and institutional nursing. This hides how low general duty nurses' salaries were.

16. E. M. Bluestone, "Introducing the Nurse to Society," *The Trained Nurse and Hospital Review* 120 (February 1948): 127 (hereafter cited as TNHR); Eli Ginzberg, "Perspectives on Nursing," AJN 47 (July 1947): 475; and "Hospital Personnel Shortage," TNHR 116 (March 1946): 180; "A Single Spirit and Purpose," TNHR 116

(May 1946): 345; "Editorials: Hospital Patients Need Nurses Now," AJN 46 (March 1946): 151.

17. Hicks, "Hospital Personnel," 179–82; "A Single Spirit," 343–46; "Nursing Shortages Can Be Overcome," TNHR 117 (May 1946): 34–37.

18. Janet M. Geister, "Candid Comments-Tomorrow Begins Today," *R.N.* 11, no. 11 (August 1948): 35; Hicks, "Hospital Personnel," 181.

19. Norman Metzger and Dennis Pointer, *Labor-Management Relations in the Health Services Industry: Theory and Practice* (Washington, D.C.: Science & Health Publications, 1972), 12–13.

20. Lieutenant, "Debits and Credits: Outline for Nursing," *R.N.* 8, no. 4 (January 1945): 8; Sutter, "Salaries," 328; Bready, "The Reason?," 706.

21. *Proceedings of the 35th Biennial Convention of the American Nurses' Association* (New York: American Nurses' Association, 1946), 13; "The Biennial," AJN 46 (November 1946): 729; Z. Lornie, "Debits and Credits: Platform," *R.N.* 10, no. 1 (October 1946): 7; R.N., "Debits and Credits: Only Human," R.N. 10, no. 1 (October 1946): 8; M. L. Paulding, "Debits and Credits: Dollar Diplomacy," *R.N.* 9, no. 4 (January 1946) 18; Bready, "The Reason?," 706; Jennie E. Strand, "Debits and Credits: Toward the Future," *R.N.* 8, no. 8 (May 1945): 7.

22. Bready, "The Reason?," 706.

23. Florence Brannigan, "The Hospital Nurse Speaks Up," TNHR 116, (January 1946): 36; Bready, "The Reason?," 706; J.C.M., "Letters-Pro and Con: Nurses' Hours," AJN 47 (July 1947): 491.

24. Alice R. Clarke, "R.N. Speaks: Where Are We Going?," *R.N.* 10, no. 8 (May 1947): 29.

25. U.S. Department of Labor, *Economic Status,* 48.

26. U.S. Department of Labor, *Economic Status,* 48.

27. Lornie, "Platform," 7–8; R.N., "Debits and Credits: Dissatisfaction," *R.N.* 10 no. 11 (November 1946): 14; Lieutenant, "Outline for Nursing," 8; "Debits and Credits: 'To Err Is Human'," *R.N.* 10, no. 7 (April 1947): 10, 12; Bernadette M. Grammont, "Debits and Credits: Double Duty," *R.N.* 10, no. 7 (April 1947): 8, 10; Lottie A. Morford, "Debits and Credits: Perils of Palmer," *R.N.* 11, no. 6 (March 1948): 14, 16; Ruth P. Topper, "Letters-Pro and Con: Happy to Be a Nurse," AJN 47 (May 1947): 337; Beverly W. White, "The General Duty Nurse Considers Her Job and Herself," AJN 46 (May 1946): 300–1.

28. Helen G. Fraser, "Debits and Credits: Urgent Needs," *R.N.* 10, no. 1 (October 1946): 14; S.M., "Letters-Pro and Con: Nursing Versus Marriage," AJN 47 (April 1947): 255; Lieutenant, "Debits and Credits: Outline for Nursing," 8.

29. U.S. Department of Labor, *Economic Status,* 18.

30. "We Can't Help Wondering" AJN 46 (November 1946): 726.

31. White, "General Duty Nurse," 300.

32. U.S. Department of Commerce, *Bureau of the Census, Historical Statistics of the United States: Colonial Times to 1970* (Washington, D.C.: U.S. Government Printing Office, 1975), D830-60; U.S. Department of Labor, *Economic Status,* 52.

33. "Personnel Policies," AJN 45 (August 1945): 593.

34. Alice Kessler-Harris, *Out to Work: A History of Wage Earning Women in the United States* (New York: Oxford Press, 1982), 264.

35. Mildred Marker, "From Our Mail Bag: 'Broken Hours,'" TNHR 115 (November 1945): 310; Florence L. McQuillan, "We Need Standards of Nursing Care," AJN 47 (February 1947): 79; U.S. Department of Labor, *Economic Status,* 21.

36. McQuillan, "We Need Standards," 79; White, "General Duty Nurse," 301; Bready, "The Reason?" 706.

37. U.S. Department of Labor, *Economic Status,* 24-25.

38. U.S. Department of Labor, *Economic Status,* 21, 23.

39. Janet M. Geister, "Candid Comments-Let's Talk It Over," *R.N.* 11, no. 7 (April 1948): 30; Geister, "Tomorrow Begins Today," 35; "Hospital Patients Need," 151.

40. McQuillan, "We Need Standards," 79; R.N., "Letters-Pro and Con: Responsibility," AJN 47 (June 1947): 418.

41. Geister, "Tomorrow Begins Today," 35.

42. Brannigan, "Hospital Nurse," 36; Signe S. Cooper, "Debits and Credits: Vindication," *R.N.* 10, no. 1 (October 1946): 10; Re-enlisted R.N. "From Our Mail Bag," TNHR 116 (May 1946): 326; R.N. "Debits and Credits: Unwanted," *R.N.* 10, no. 9 (June 1947): 8.

43 Ex-Army R.N., "From Our Mailbag," TNHR 116 (May 1946): 326; Edith M. F. Pritchard, "National Nursing Now," TNHR 117(December 1946): 418; Brannigan, "Why Army Nurses," 56.

44. Bertha W. Mears, "The Forty Hour Week! but How?" AJN 47 (January 1947): 8.

45. "31,000 Army Nurses and Their Post-War Plans," AJN 45 (December 1945): 1021.

46. Brown, *Nursing for the Future,* 46–47; Everett C. Hughes et al.*Twenty Thousand Nurses Tell Their Story* (Philadelphia: J. B. Lippincott, 1958), 72, 168.

47. Janet M. Geister, "Plain talk." NHR, 114, (April 1945): 276–78; R.N., "From Our Mail Bag," TNHR 115, (December 1945): 392.

48. Brown, *Nursing for the Future,* 46–47; Kathryn Cahill, "Debits and Credits: M.D. vs. R.N.," *R.N.* 9, no. 7 (April 1946): 7–8; "Hospital Patients Need," 151.

49. Brown, *Nursing for the Future,* 47.

50. "Editorials: What's Really Back of the Nursing Shortage?" *New York Medicine,* 2, no. 18 (20 September 1946): 11.

51. Brown, *Nursing for the Future,* 45, 54.

52. U.S. Department of Labor, *Economic Status,* 1.

53. Loraine Himel, "Debits and Credits: Pursuit of Happiness," *R.N.* 11, no. 11 (August, 1948): 7

54. Chafe, *Paradox of Change,* 121-34; Evans, *Born to Liberty,* 22, 208, 219–29; Hartmann, *Home Front,* 20–21.

55. Chafe, *Paradox of Change,* 154–72; Evans, *Born to Liberty,* 229–34; Hartmann, *Home Front,* 23–27; May, *Homeward Bound,* 58–77.

56. Chafe, *Paradox of Change,* 166.

57. Chafe, *Paradox of Change,* 158–63; Kessler-Harris, *Out to Work,* 299, 300–303; Evans, *Born for Liberty,* 250–55.

58. Theresa I. Lynch, "Recruitment - 1951," AJN 52 (March 1952): 301–3; "How Many Will Choose Nursing?," AJN 55 (October 1955): 1195.

59. U.S. Department of Labor, *Economic Status*, 54; Ester L. Middlewood, "Why Do Students Drop Out?," AJN 46 (December 1946): 838–40.

60. American Nurses' Association, *Facts About Nursing, 1950*, (New York: Author, 1950), 35 (hereafter cited as ANA). This decline reflects the end of the U.S. Cadet Nurse Corps in June 1995, Philip A. Kalisch and Beatrice J. Kalisch, *The Advancement of American Nursing*, 23rd ed. (Boston: Little, Brown, 1995), 341.

61. In the eleven years prior to this, nursing school enrollments were increasing steadily from 67,533 in 1935, to 91,457 in 1941, and to 126,576 in 1945, ANA, *Facts About Nursing, 1945* (New York: Author, 1945), 34; ANA, *Facts About Nursing*, 35.

62. ANA, *Facts About Nursing: A statistical summary, 1959* (New York: Author, 1959), 7.

63. Eugenia Kaledin, *American Women in the 1950s, Mothers and More* (Boston: Twayne Publishers, 1984), Preface.

64. "They Chose Nursing Thoughtfully," AJN 48 (February, 1948): 80–81; Himel, "Pursuit of Happiness," 7–8; R.N., "Debits and Credits: The Happy Side," *R.N.* 9, no. 8 (May, 1946): 7; M.B., "Letters-Pro and Con: Kindliness," AJN 47 (June 1947): 418; Ellwynne M. Vreeland, "Why Do Nurses Nurse?," AJN 49 (July 1949): 412–13.

65. M. B., "Kindliness," 418.

66. "They Chose Nursing Thougtfully," 80.

67. "They Chose Nursing Thougtfully," 80–81; Vreeland, "Why Do Nurses Nurse?," 412; Theodora Sharrocks, "Nursing is Great Experience," AJN 47 (February 1947): 81; Edna S. Moody, "I'm Glad I'm a Nurse," AJN 47 (February 1947): 79–80; R.N., "The Happy Side," 7.

68. Dora Lewenstein, "Letters-Pro and Con: Professional Ideals and Practical Problems," AJN 47 (March 1947): 186; Gretta Palmer, "What Happens When Trained Nurses Won't Nurse the Sick?" *R.N.* 11, no. 4 (January 1948): 48–51, 68–70, 73, 74, 76–78.

69. Ben Olds and Dan Herr, "Where's That Nurse?" *The Saturday Evening Post*, 4 January 1947, p. 17, 81–82; Palmer, "What Happens," 48-49; Howard Whitman and Douglas Ingells, "Don't Curse the Nurse," *Collier* 119 (31 May 1947): 26, 67-69.

70. Palmer, "What Happens," 48–51, 68–70, 73, 74, 76–78.

71. Alice R. Clarke, "R.N. Speaks: Nursing, the Stormy Petrel" *R.N.* 11, no. 4 (January 1948): 32–33, 82, 84; Hester Manatt, "Debits and Credits: Perils of Palmer," *R.N.* 11, no. 6 (March 1948): 14; Lottie A. Morford, "Debits and Credits: Perils of Palmer," *R.N.* 11, no. 6 (March 1948): 14–16; R.N., "Debits and Credits: Perils of Palmer," *R.N.* 11, no. 6 (March 1948): 18; Bernard V. Bowen, "Debits and Credits: Perils of Palmer," *R.N.* 11, no. 6 (March 1948): 18.

72. Mary R. Shelton, "We Can Help," AJN 49 (July 1949): 413.

73. Chafe, *The Paradox of Change*, 153–93; May, *Homeward Bound*, 159–61.

74. Shelton, "We Can Help," 413.

75. Hicks, "Hospital Personnel" 178; Janet M. Geister, "Candid Comments-Lets talk It Over," *R.N.* 11, no. 7 (April 1948), 28–31.

76. Brown, *Nursing for the Future*, 47; Janet M. Geister,. "The Hospital and the Nurse," *The Modern Hospital* 89, no. 2 (August 1948): 59–61.

77. Brown, *Nursing for the Future*, 47; Shirley Titus, "Economic Facts of Life for Nurses: I," AIN 52 (1952): 1110.

78. Titus, "Economic Facts," 1110.

79. Victoria T. Grando, "ANA's Economic Security Program: The First 20 Years," *Nursing Research* 46 (1997): 111–15.

80. Victoria T. Grando, "Nurses' Struggle for Economic Equity: 1945 to 1965," in *Dissertation Abstracts International University* (Ann Arbor: University, Microfilms International, 1994), p. 224, 9504017.

BOOK REVIEWS

American Medicine and the Public Interest:
A History of Specialization
By Rosemary Stevens
(Berkeley, Calif.: University of California Press, 1998)

Rosemary Stevens's pathbreaking 1971 study of medical specialization and its consequences for health care and public policy in the United States has been republished by the University of California Press with a new introduction and updated bibliography. The reappearance of the work is welcome. Carefully and prodigiously researched, it is an indispensable reference which offers a rich and detailed account—541 pages worth—of the "specialized, disorganized, expansionary, and flamboyant" (p. 9) American medical profession in the first seven decades of this century. And, save for "confident predictions that national health insurance was around the corner" (p. 19), Stevens's assessment of the profession and the private, entrepreneurial culture which sustained it, are as insightful and helpful today as they were nearly 30 years ago.

The introduction to the updated edition has utility as well. Here Stevens reviews recent scholarship in the medical profession, medical institutions, and the politics of health care in America, evaluates her work in light of it, and underscores the continuing relevance of the query at the heart of American Medicine and the Public Interest: "what is, and what should be, the relationship of the profession of medicine and the public interest?" (p. 19)

The answers to the question, Stevens makes clear, are intimately related to specialization, "*the* fundamental theme for the organization of medicine in the twentieth century" (p. ix). Initially prompted by scientific advances in medicine, specialization grew rapidly in response to such disparate factors as physician opposition to fee-splitting, a tradition of antielitism in the profession, hospital expansion, war, and federal subsidy of medical research. Inevitably, specialty organizations emerged, e.g., the American College of Surgeons (1910), and the American College of Physicians (1915), along with specialty boards designed to "certify" practitioners. A specialty board surely of interest to nurse historians and nurse anesthetists is the American Board of Anesthesiology, founded in 1937. Unfortunately, Stevens offers only a brief account of nurse anesthetists and their role in the decision of physician anesthesiologists to establish a board to assure specialist identification and certification. Here, and in the analysis of the hospital's place in the history of specialization, Stevens would do well to accord more attention to nurses and nursing.

Nursing History Review 8 (2000): 185-212. A publication of the American Association for the History of Nursing. Copyright © 2000 Springer Publishing Company.

Today, Stevens reports, there are 24 specialty boards and "a byzantine array of certifying programs (p. 25)." The American Board of Medical Specialties listed "37 general areas of certification plus 75 subspecialties in 1997"; the American Medical Association identified "78 distinct types of specialty and subspecialty residency programs in 1996" (p. 25). Thus has the profession of medicine established a relationship with the American public: the "public interest" and what it "should be" are other matters altogether. Indeed, the meaning and consequences of specialization and a private and self-interested certification process for public policy and patient care, Stevens reveals, were issues little regarded by the specialty groups, by the American Medical Association, or other national medical organizations. Their failure to consider the public interest is reflected in the American Medical Association's opposition to national health insurance proposals from the 1930s on, and in specialists' self-serving approach to Medicare reimbursement before the advent of DRGs.

In her discussion of Medicare and other federal efforts to promote health care programs in the public interest, Stevens is as thorough, thoughtful, and judicious as she is in her analysis of the development of America's specialized medical profession. In consequence, historians interested in 20th-century nursing will find *American Medicine and the Public Interest* a rich resource, an invaluable introduction to the "special world" in which nurses practiced in the period. Not incidentally, Stevens's account of medicine's specialization is also a useful cautionary tale for today's nurse specialists, their "certifying" organizations, and the American Nurses Association in its continuing efforts to bring coherence and clarity to credentialing in advanced practice nursing.

JUDITH M. STANLEY, PHD
Professor of History
California State University, Hayward
25800 Carlos Bee Blvd.
Hayward, CA 94542

Bedside Seductions: Nursing and the Victorian Imagination, 1830-1880

By Catherine Judd
(New York: St. Martin's Press, 1998)

You can't tell a book by its title, or can you? Asked to write the foreword, many years ago, for that well-known illustrated history of nursing, I was concerned about its title, *Nursing, the Oldest Art*. Apparently I was not alone in my concern, for by the time the book reached the bookstores it was entitled,

Nursing, the Finest Art. All this is by way of saying you could be misled or your expectations unfulfilled by the title of this book—*Bedside Seductions: Nursing and the Victorian Imagination, 1830-1880.*

Knowing that the author teaches 19th-century British Literature and Women's Studies may help prepare you. For you will become acquainted with topics such as "Social Healing and the Pathology of the Victorian Novel"; "Nursing, Sexuality and the Dangerous Classes"; Nursing and the Carceral in *Jane Eyre;* and "Metaphors of Female Artistry in Gaskell's Ruth." If you manage to work through these four chapters then you will be rewarded.

For it is in chapter 5, "A Female Ulysses: Mary Seacole, Homeric Epic and the Trope of Heroic Nursing (1854-1857), that Judd's presentation of history strikes a welcome balance with literature. This chapter informs and satisfies!

The author promises from the beginning that what will be demonstrated is the transformation of ". . . the humble sickroom attendant of the late eighteenth century . . . into a pivotal cultural icon of the Mid -Victorian era" (p. xii).

Using literature and social history for her framework, Judd explains the importance of the nurse ". . . as a paradigm for imaginary resolutions to ideological problems faced by Mid-Victorians" (p. 2). She states her purpose is ". . . to set in motion the hitherto inert and typologizing classification of the Victorian nurse through their reinsertion into a concrete historical situation" (p. 2). In other words, the years 1830-1873 will provide the time frame, the context will be provided by literary examples which may or may not be familiar to readers of NHR. Along the way there is the hope that an explanation of the traditional attribution of sexuality to nursing will be evident.

Strangely enough, the author begins chapter 5 by analyzing a painting, "The Nurse" by Sir Lawrence Alma-Tadema (1872). Her interpretation of this painting apparently is meant to set the stage but in truth serves only to cast doubt, as art interpretation is tricky and in this instance was not convincing and seemed superfluous.

By the time Mary Seacole is introduced the reader is ready and pleasantly impressed with both the historical and literary contexts that are developed. Seacole becomes larger than life and at the same time convincingly real as a Crimean heroine.

In the last chapter, literature and nursing, personified by George Eliot and Florence Nightingale, are brought full circle. Yet Judd reminds us that ". . . Nightingale was primarily a writer, her literal manifestation as a nurse spanning only a few years of her sixty-odd-year career" (p. 130). The information that follows provides a curious view of two dynamic women who were active social reformers with similar backgrounds and interests. According to Judd, they both sought altruistic satisfaction, and traveled in the same social circles, but competition was very much in evidence in their individual quest for intellectual, spiritual and vocational recognition.

Although the book comes to an abrupt end, Judd's promise for the last chapter was ". . . to investigate the intersection of science and sentiment conveyed by the figure of the nurse, and the ways . . . this convergence helped

. . . create . . . parallel and competing theories"(p. 15) as they relate to female social leadership. In the final analysis her argument is an engaging one. For Judd, the ". . . subtle convergence between the militancy of the Nightingale nurse and the humanitarian sympathy embodied in Eliot's nursing persona" (p. 121) provides the reader with the best of both worlds.

OLGA MARANJIAN CHURCH, PhD, FAAN
Professor, University of Connecticut
Storrs, CT 06269

Virginia Avenel Henderson: Signature for Nursing
Edited by Eleanor Krohn Herrmann
(Indianapolis, Ind.: Sigma Theta Tau, 1998)

Characterized as a *Festschrift* by its editor and publisher, this book is a delightful read! Its purpose is to describe and honor one of nursing's legends, Virginia A. Henderson, who died 19 March 1996, at the age of 98. Publication coincides with the 100th anniversary of her birth (30 November 1897).

The book comprises 35 short (2-4 pages) chapters or testimonials, each of which describes Henderson from the perspective or experience of the author. These chapters are organized into three parts: leadership, scholarship, and humanitarianism.

Each testimonial offers a unique glimpse of Henderson's thinking, personality, habits, likes, and dislikes. Her spirit and human qualities are so well described that after reading only a few testimonials, one begins to feel that one knows her, or is talking with her. Right away, a strong sense of her personality and "essence" emerges, and this character portrait gains added substance from the information on Henderson's accomplishments and influence on nursing found in the remainder of the book. Anyone familiar with Henderson and her work will be able to proceed smoothly through the book and feel like they had just read a full biography. Although it was not written for use as historical documentation, the book features many interesting historical tidbits (for example, how Henderson got fired from Teachers College).

The variety of people who contributed to the book makes it exceptional. While esteemed colleagues, precious friends, and loyal family members are naturally included, less well-known people also share their thoughts. These include Henderson's minister, physician, hospice nurse and a young woman who first met her as a child when invited to be a hostess at a party. Some of the relationships date back to the 1930s, while others were in existence for only a few months.

The book is well written in a consistent style even though it has 37 individual contributors, and this is the mark of good editing on Herrmann's part. There are appendices that contain biographical notes and list major awards, honorary degrees, and honorary associations. The appendices could have been expanded to include publications and organizational contributions, but this is a minor criticism of a book which should have wide appeal.

LAURIE K. GLASS, RN, PhD, FAAN
Professor and Director, Center for Nursing History
University of Wisconsin-Milwaukee School of Nursing
P.O. Box 413
Milwaukee, WI 53201-0413

Critical Care Nursing: A History

By Julie Fairman & Joan Lynaugh
(Philadelphia: University of Pennsylvania Press 1998)

Critical Care Nursing: A History explores the development of critical care nursing in the United States between 1950 and 1970. The authors, Joan Lynaugh and Julie Fairman study the rise of critical care nursing using a social history framework. They tell a compelling story about the development of this specialization through the vantage point of the participants who helped create it. Interviews with nurses and physicians, accounts written during the 1940s-1990s, records of Chestnut Hill Hospital and the Hospital of the University of Pennsylvania, and other social histories about nursing provide the references from which the story emerges. The book is organized into six chapters that define critical care nursing, describe the transitions hospitals underwent during the post-World War II period, explore the changes nurses experienced in practice, education, and professional development, portray the complex negotiations between nurses and physicians during these transitions, depict the rise of specialty organizations in nursing, and reflect on the ethical and moral dimensions of critical care at the end of the 20th century.

The definition of critical care includes two very important but competing constructs that are essential to understanding the history of this specialty. The notion that a patient must be in a physiologically unstable condition and in danger of dying sharply contrasts with the expectation that critical care nursing was targeted for those expected to live. The authors offer a penetrating analysis of critical care nursing, framing the collected stories and excellent documentation within this competing construct. The nursing care received by the gravely ill patient, who with care is expected to live, is framed against the backdrop of the changing hospital, developing professional roles, scientific discoveries, and economic constraints.

The authors direct us to look at nursing history for the origin of critical care. Nurses have traditionally provided lifesaving measures through careful observation of the patient. At different times in nursing's history, triage of the sick and wounded called for the grouping of seriously ill patients for care. As an example, the authors present Louisa Mae Alcott's 1863 description of three distinct patient groups requiring different levels of nursing care. Florence Nightingale called for triage of the wounded and sick. The changes in technology and the provision of emergency care during World War II and the Korean War led the public to expect similar kinds of treatment for the civilian population. The successful use of antibiotics decreased the number of people hospitalized with infectious diseases thereby increasing the number of people hospitalized for cardiovascular diseases and the like. The staffing shortages and architectural changes in hospitals placed the critical care patient at greater risk. The underlying fundamental concept of hospitals, to offer "safe, efficient, and humane" care for the sick, provided the impetus for hospitals to pay for the nursing care needed.

Although not a new concept in nursing, the establishment of critical care units where expert nurses learn and practice their art was a result of the transition that hospitals experienced in the 1950s, 1960s and 1970s. An increase in complexity of illness and new methods with which to save lives increased the likelihood of successful patient outcomes. Furthermore, the combination of these events, coupled with the changes in nursing education and the changing role of women, contributed to the rise of this new specialty in nursing. Establishment of trusting, professional relationships that redefined roles and responsibilities between nurses and physicians contributed to the development of the critical care units. Despite the initial concern expressed by hospital boards for the high cost, the increased knowledge and collaboration needed between professionals, and the grouping of male and female critically ill patients together, critical care units proliferated at an exceptional rate and became firmly established in health care history.

Critical Care Nursing provides an outstanding critique of critical care nursing in six, concisely written chapters. It provides us with insights that are useful for educators, clinicians, historians and anyone interested in nursing, medicine, and health care. The book includes photographs that provide an excellent visual contextual framework. The organizational history of the American Association of Critical-Care Nurses (AACN), and the contribution it has made to this specialty is particularly enlightening and important. The book not only is scholarly written and well-referenced, but is a pleasure to read, easy to follow, and one that is highly recommended.

SANDRA BETH LEWENSON, PhD, RN

Associate Professor of Nursing
Associate Dean, Department of Graduate Studies
Pace University
Lienhard School of Nursing
861 Bedford Road
Pleasantville, NY 10570

Alaska's Search for a Killer:
A Seafaring Medical Adventure, 1946-1948
By Susan Meredith
(Juneau, Alaska Public Health Nursing History Association, 1998)

In *On The Teaching & Writing of History* (1994), Bernard Bailyn is asked "What distinctions do you make between history and biography, both of which focus upon activity or subject matter of the past?" (p. 77). In answer he paraphrases Paul Lazarsfeld, equating biography and autobiography, and gives the three justifications for biography being a piece of history. The first is that the person is of great consequence in human affairs, the second that the person is representative of a particular group important in human affairs and the third is that the person is an excellent witness. He states, "Although they may not have been representative of anything in particular and certainly did not shape history, they were present at the right place and the right time" (p. 78). Susan Meredith, the author of *Alaska's Search for a Killer,* is such a witness.

This detailed narrative in diary format tells the story of the *MV Hygiene,* a floating health clinic launched by the Alaskan Territorial Department of Health to attack an epidemic of TB between 1946 and 1948. The time is crucial in American history, American Public Health history and that of the development of the state of Alaska. Susan Meredith, a young bacteriologist, tells this tale in a personal manner using both chronology and geography as an organizing framework. I found reading this work intriguing, for not only does it shed light on the inner workings of a frontline public health team fighting a tragic disease, but also because it reveals how geography influences human activity. The author uses geography in the manner suggested by W. Gordon East (1965) not only as topography, but also as the everyday physical environment and the intermittent dramatic episodes of weather in descriptions as a significant factor influencing the populace and the mission *MV Hygiene.* She provides vivid descriptions of how geography affected individual residents and visitors, the structure of local communities and cultures, the operations of the health team, and life aboard ship.

This is also a tale of adventure in the Alaskan wilderness, and of the courage and commitment of the author, the nurse, and other members of the *Hygiene* team. Meredith describes the challenges of recording the scope of the TB epidemic and its devastation among Alaskan native populations. In addition, her diary reveals the consequences of poor therapeutic alternatives, disruptive team members, and the rapid turnover of personnel within the context of constant movement along the often beautiful yet stark Alaskan coast.

Closely allied with the nurse assigned to the team, the author (cross-trained as an x-ray technologist) examines firsthand the health concerns of various local populations, and the strength and weaknesses of team members and their roles. The team nurse and her nursing colleagues assigned to remote areas are frequently viewed as necessary for team effectiveness. Nurses and teachers are seen as the facilitators of health care delivery and local community use of "modern resources" to improve the lives of isolated peoples. Teachers in remote communities appear as the natural allies of the nurses in meeting basic human needs for adequate nutrition, sanitation, protection from the harsh environment, and basic health care. Commentary on relationships between the team and the various physicians assigned to the *Hygiene* is reminiscent of the conflicts in today's acute care teams. Gender, race, professional positions, politics, and the structure and lack of financial depth of the Territorial Health Department all play roles in this tale of a war against a killer disease. Big business interests (fishing and canning) and government (U.S. Congress treatment of Alaska as a territory and military installations) are explored in terms of their effects on the native populations and the environment.

Susan Meredith, with the assistance of Kitty Gair (nurse on the *MV Hygiene*) and Elaine Schwinge (physician for a rotation on the *MV Hygiene*), uses diaries, letters, official reports, and personal reflections to reconstruct this post-WWII experience. Although describing a public health team's experience grounded by the time, place and the structure of its mission, this historical reflection provides insights into a variety of situations nurses have faced and will face again in attempting to work collaboratively to meet patient needs.

Alaska's Search for a Killer will appeal to historians interested in Alaska's development, public health, nursing, and geography as a framework for studying human activity. In addition, this is also a fairly entertaining adventure story for students of public health nursing, or those interested in Alaska and its vast seacoast.

References

Bailyn, B. 1994. *On The Teaching & Writing of History*. Hanover, NH: University Press of New England.

East, W. G. 1965. *The Geography Behind History*. New York: W. W. Norton & Co.

ELIZABETH A. TROUGHT PhD, RN
430 Baywood Drive
Winterville, NC 28590

Purity and Pollution:
Gender, Embodiment, and Victorian Medicine
By Alison Bashford
(New York: St. Martin's Press, 1998)

The cover photograph of a Victorian operating theater gives the reader a tantalizing invitation to this erudite text. A neat and tidy nurse stands at attention next to a dormant patient on an operating table, surrounded by two gowned physicians and an anesthetist in shirtsleeves. Immediately the reader wonders why the female nurse is the image of cleanliness, in contrast to the others. The author answers this question in an expository introduction, setting up a framework of gender and social theory, sturdily supported by primary source material, that runs through the book. The works of other scholars in gender, social, and medical history are quoted, commented on, and enlarged by her new interpretations.

Industrialization and urbanization precipitated the public health and sanitary reform movements of the 1800s, for they brought the dirt and filth that were recognized as unhealthy. Victorian culture associated order and cleanliness with purity, uncleanness with pollution. Purity and cleanliness implied morality, while pollution and uncleanness suggested its opposite, immorality. Thus, moral reform came to be epitomized in the age-old adage that "cleanliness is next to godliness."

Domestic spaces were the first area for sanitary reform, so it is natural that women took on responsibilities for carrying out sanitary practices. Bashford notes that this led to middle- and upper-class women gaining authority in the public health movement. She shows that this authority also depended on their elevated social status within a philanthropic Victorian culture. The author argues that it was a small step, then, to socially transfer women's authority over domestic sanitation to hospital spaces where women, in the form of female nurses, were managed by women of social status, i.e., nurse superintendents. Physicians and influential figures, Florence Nightingale not the least of them, promoted sanitary reform at every turn. Nightingale's political activities, writings on sanitation of sick rooms and hospitals, and the St. Thomas training program all revolve around sanitation practices. The author offers an interesting discussion on how Nightingale could refuse to accept the reductionistic germ theory and still believe that dirt and pollution were themselves responsible for illness. This discussion should be of particular interest to nurses.

The next three chapters explore and discuss the cultural reconfiguration of the nurse, how sexual attitudes and religious values influenced the discipline of nursing, and how physicians became pathologized by puerperal fever in the 1860s. The balance of the book examines female medical practitioners in light of shifts in gendered politics in medicine, the social obstacles associated with women dissecting dead bodies, and sepsis and asepsis in relation to gender. Even though the primary focus of research is England, Bashford's analyses may be considered valid for other countries that looked to England as their chief sociocultural influence.

The author places physicians, nurses, and women side by side in her theoretical framework and interpretations, believing that the evolution of one cannot be considered without the others. The text is the richer for this conviction. Across its range of topics, *Purity and Pollution* is interesting, scholarly, and worthy of serious consideration. Bashford's effective narrative style speaks to the reader as if the two were engaged in conversation across a seminar table. She achieves the goal of the true historical researcher: overturning prior knowledge by reforming it with valid new information, thus presenting innovative historical perspectives. By shining the light of other academic disciplines and theories upon our own, the author illuminates connections and relationships that deepen our understanding of nursing history.

SANDRA KRESS DAVIS, EdD, RN
Adjunct Faculty, School of Nursing
La Salle University
3652 Haywood St.
Philadelphia, PA 19129-1531

Mothers and Motherhood: Readings in American History
Edited by Rima D. Apple and Janet Golden
(Columbus: Ohio State University Press, 1997)

The articles included in *Mothers and Motherhood* weave a story of American women who over the course of time have both challenged and accepted prevailing social, political, and economic norms of mothering. The conceptions of mothers and motherhood range from Mary Palmer Tyler's view of citizenship for women in a new republic, to the struggle of slave women for respect as mothers, to immigrant women's abilities to adapt to American ideas, and finally to the late 20th-century welfare debate for female-headed families. The authors included in this compilation together form a diversity of views that gives the reader a broad perspective on the experiences and perceptions of and by mothers.

The book is organized into four sections. The first section looks at the social construction of motherhood. The seven articles included in this section illustrate the changing definitions and meanings of mothers and motherhood to the mothers themselves and to society at large. The articles range from an analysis of the cultural significance of breast-feeding in the 17th and 18th centuries to the construction of "proper" motherhood in the Emmett Till civil rights case of the 1950s. A focus on emotion is found throughout the articles, especially in one dealing with mother love in the 19th century and another describing maternal grief as seen through the pages of *True Story*, a periodical with a largely White, working-class readership. An article on motherhood and the practice of wet nursing also demonstrates the influence of emotion on mothers' lives.

The second section discusses motherhood and reproduction. Midwifery, birth control in the 18th and 19th centuries, infertility, anaesthetized deliveries, African American women and abortion, and alternative births are discussed. While different, these articles demonstrate that all women, regardless of the path to (or from) reproduction they take, share common problems and triumphs along the way.

The third section looks at social and cultural settings for mothers and motherhood. Racial, ethnic, and cultural differences in various settings are discussed and the ways these differences dictate mothering practices are analyzed. Slave mothers in the Antebellum South, Irish American mothers and single women in the late 19th and early 20th centuries, Jewish mothers and immigrant daughters in the 1920s and 30s, and Japanese American mothers from 1940 to 1990 are described and analyzed. In addition, articles on mothers in the La Lèche League in the late 1950s through the 1980s and on the similarities and differences in motherhood practices among Black and White women involved in women's liberation ideology during the 1960s lend a more contemporary feel to the discussion and demonstrate that social and cultural settings continue to influence mothers and motherhood in our own times.

The final section of the book deals with public policy and motherhood. The articles included discuss the ways official agencies utilized mothers to further not so hidden agendas. To Americanize Mexican immigrants, government agencies established programs aimed at mothers or potential mothers, believing mothers the key to the family. Between 1910 and 1930 Illinois public health officials teamed with rural mothers to reform health for families originally felt to be better off than their city counterparts. The Roosevelt and subsequent administrations have sought, but ultimately failed, to legally abolish industrial homework. Both sides in this debate have used mothers and the concept of motherhood to illustrate the pros and cons of this type of work. Other articles discuss and analyze the work of the National Congress of Mothers, the beginnings of feminist birth control ideas in the late 19th century, and the evolution of welfare and mandatory wage earning for female welfare recipients in the 20th century.

Apple and Golden have chosen articles for this volume that provide a focus on the influence of American society on mothers and motherhood since the colonial era. The articles clearly demonstrate that motherhood means more than bearing and raising a child. The organization of the book into four sections allows the reader to understand these different meanings without difficulty. The editors' introductions to the four sections help to draw together the major issues and ideologies represented by the articles. For these reasons, this fascinating look at one of the major roles for women in our society should be of interest to anyone interested in women's history or American history in general.

ELIZABETH A. WALSH REEDY
Doctoral Candidate
School of Nursing
University of Pennsylvania
Philadelphia, PA 19104

Nursing History and the Politics of Welfare
Edited by Anne Marie Rafferty, Jane Robinson, and Ruth Elkan
(London and New York: Routledge, 1997)

Originally presented at the first *Nursing History and the Politics of Welfare* Conference at the University of Nottingham in 1993, the 15 papers in this edited book address the pervasive influence of societal, cultural, economic, and political factors, as well as components of Nightingale's legacy, on the welfare of nurses and recipients of nursing care.

In the first chapter, the reader is confronted by Steppe's poignant description of "one of the darkest chapters in the history of nursing," as she recounts the socioeconomic, political, and obedience-conformist influences that prompted German nurses to carry out Nazi "health" policies. In South Africa, gender and race were evident in employment practices in the late 18th and early 19th centuries when, as detailed by Deacon in chapter 5, colonial and government practices continued the long tradition of using White women as nurses at the Robben Island leper hospital and mental asylum, even when they were untrained nurses and the practice was contrary to general procedures. Although professional nursing had become a prestigious occupation for African women in the 20th century, Marks notes, in chapter 2, the continuing dualisms in South African health services, such as superior doctors and inferior nurses, feminine caring and male rationality, and divisions between Black and White personnel.

Unintended outcomes of the Rockefeller health campaign in the Philippines are examined by Brush in chapter 3. An agenda of colonialism and decades of nursing education, focused on western standards and hospital-based care rather than community health practice, resulted in an oversupply of nurses with hospital technical skills but lacking the skills to address the public health needs of the indigenous Philippine population. Alternatively, Fitzgerald, in chapter 4, ascribes a greater cultural understanding to the female medical missionaries in their care of women in Colonial India.

Australia is the focus of chapters 6, 10, and 11. In an analysis of 19th century caregiving by convicts, Cushing contends that the popular conception of female convicts as immoral, perpetuated by the paternalism and chauvinism of the era, was unwarranted, and credits Nightingale's reforms for improvements in caregiving and the image of women. However, a few decades later, economic conditions for nurses declined and compared unfavorably to that of other workers. Godden explains how a public debate found politicians and the general public in favor of better hours and wages for nurses, while nurse leaders held to Nightingale's belief that nursing was organized philanthropy and long hours were intrinsic to nursing. Even when a severe nursing shortage prevailed during World War II, nurses' salaries and conditions of work were not improved. Strachan speculates on reasons why the government attempted to staff hospitals by force rather than raising salaries, despite many entreaties to do so.

Mortimer paints a brighter picture of social and economic success in chapter 7. Through gaining the confidence of doctors and clients, domiciliary nurses in mid-19th-century England were able to establish a way of living as independent women. Abrams, in chapter 12, explores the Rockefeller Foundation's ambivalence over nursing leaders' attempt to define nursing's jurisdiction based on issues of power and gender.

In chapters 8 and 9, Olson and Bioschama, respectively, question caring and holism as concepts basic to nursing. From a feminine perspective, caring makes intuitive sense but masculine traits, such as controlling and managing, are necessary traits of female nurses. And whereas holism was cited as relevant to public health nursing, it is, in many ways, incompatible with nursing in hospitals that stress technology and efficiency.

Baer vigorously challenges the "equal" stance of many feminists in chapter 14. She rejects the feminist practice of rewarding and supporting women who take on the work of men, while talented women in work traditionally designated as feminine are neither honored nor supported. She also calls for linguistic changes in terms such as health care instead of medical care, and patient treatment plans rather than doctor's orders. In chapter 13 Maxwell examines the relationship between social work and health visiting by nurses with children and families in England, and cites such collaborative work as essential to the welfare of families. The last chapter, by Hall, discusses nursing's need for more archival repositories.

Readers concerned with nursing's special contributions to health care and the realities of the politics of welfare will benefit from reading these insightful historical analyses that reflect on a mix of feminist and social perspectives. The various authors' ideas provide ample food for thought for those considering the opportunities and challenges professional nursing faces in the 21st century.

GRACE P. ERICKSON, EdD, RNC
Assistant Professor
College of Nursing
University of South Florida
12901 Bruce B. Downs Blvd.
Tampa, FL 33612-4766

Alternative Health Care in Canada: Nineteenth- and Twentieth-Century Perspectives
Compiled and edited by J. K. Crellin,
R. R. Anderson, and J. T. H. Connor
(Toronto: Canadian Scholars' Press, 1997).

Kindly Medicine: Physio-Medicalism in America, 1836-1911
By John S. Haller, Jr.
(Kent, Ohio: Kent State University Press, 1997).

Populist health movements, feminism, and postmodernist world views contributed to increased consumer dissatisfaction with a technological, biomedical model of health care based on "curing." As socioeconomic and legislative forces create new opportunities in health care, nurses (who have traditionally claimed a philosophy of holistic "caring") are strategically situated for expanded roles and incorporation of alternative treatment modalities into their practice. In assuming these new roles, nurses would benefit by understanding how allopathic medicine came to dominate health care, effectively eliminating and/or limiting other therapies. *Alternative Health Care in Canada* and *Kindly Medicine* shift our frame of reference from the view of health care as a dichotomous choice (alternative versus orthodox) to understanding health care diversity within the context of social forces, economics, and ideologies.

Alternative Health Care in Canada: Nineteenth- and Twentieth-Century Perspectives is an anthology of readings compiled and edited partially in response to the needs of an interdisciplinary anthropology-sociology course in health care. Its stated purpose is to reveal "the complexity of factors both favoring and undermining roles for alternative medicine" and to examine "the ways scholarly disciplines study alternative practices." The editors present an overview of current issues interspersed with 16 readings which include four historical studies. Initially intended for classroom use in medical schools, social science courses, and medical history courses, the book also appeals to "all readers as partners with physicians in approaches to health care" and "administrators, health care professionals or anyone concerned."

Alternative health care is described as a polymorphic social movement, expanded in definition to encompass complementary medicine, holistic medicine, natural medicine, and "*médicine douce*." The range of therapies includes homeopathy, chiropractic, eclecticism, naturopathy, herbal or botanical medicine, aboriginal practices, Chinese medicine, and massage—but intentionally excludes midwifery. Questions are raised regarding practice standards, professionalization, the nature of therapy and its effectiveness, and the nature of medical knowledge in general. The editors suggest that ambiguities result when "alternatives" become accepted as orthodox practices, as "regular" and "alternative" labels shift depending on the culturally defined point of reference, and as the established professions disagree regarding accepted practice.

For historians, the strength of this book consists of the four historical studies: J.T.H. Conner's *A Sort of Felo-de-Se: Eclecticism, Related Medical Sects, and Their Decline in Victorian Ontario;* David Coburn's *State Authority, Medical Dominance, and Trends in the Regulation of the Health Professions: The Ontario Case;* Barbara Clow's, *Mahlon William Locke: 'Toe-Twister;* and E.H. Gort and D. Coburn's, *Naturopathy in Canada: Changing Relationships to Medicine, Chiropractic and the State.*

Conner uses a sociopolitical framework to examine activities of the Eclectics in Ontario, from their origins in Thomsonism to their absorption into mainstream medicine during the early 1900s. He focuses on educational, organizational, and licensing structures which shaped Eclectic practice, arguing that their "eventual demise was not wholly due to the monopolistic impulses of competing regular physicians . . ." but also to "the conscious decision of the majority of Eclectics themselves." Conner suggests this process was fundamentally different from the American process.

From a sociological perspective, Coburn studies the relationship between the state and professions, providing an overview of differences between the Canadian and American systems. His analysis of nursing was edited out, significantly limiting the usefulness for nursing history. Coburn argues that rationalization reduced medical control over health care divisions of labor and restructured both the state/professional and interprofessional relationships. Through the financing of health insurance plans and control over education, the Canadian government also shaped professional self-regulation.

Clow's research on *Mahlon William Locke, "Toe-Twister,"* makes for an excellent and fascinating read. She uses a case study approach to consider one alternative health care practice in small-town, rural Ontario between 1925 and 1942. Locke was an early 20th-century physician who incorporated the unorthodox method of foot manipulation for arthritis and other illnesses, reputedly treating over 1,000 patients per week. His burgeoning practice had a great impact on the community and on the medical profession as patients practiced "cross-border shopping" for alternative care. One result was a considerable loss of American funds to the Canadian economy during the Depression. Clow contrasts the American Medical Association's strong denouncement and activism against Locke with the Canadian responses of 'shrewd' silence, collegiality as professional protection, and reliance on governmental regulation rather than mobilization of professional or public opinion.

Gort and Coburn consider the recent reemergence of nutrition, life style counselling, and prevention in relation to the historical practice of naturopathy in Ontario during the "halcyon years" from the 1920s to the 1930s. This study uses occupational formation, professionalization, and medical dominance as analytical concepts to examine the development of naturopathy and its relationships to medicine, chiropractic, and the state.

"Editorial shortening" constitutes a significant limitation of this anthology. Readers must question the absence of nurses' voices related to alternative health care practices, given its educational mandate. Readers must also carefully discriminate between the historical research and current/popular materials included in the readings. Given these limitations, however, *Alternative Health Care in Canada* contributes to medical historiography through a timely collection of articles on a topic which has not yet been adequately researched by historians.

Kindly Medicine: Physio-Medicalism in America, 1836-1911 presents a different framework and analysis of alternative health care practice. Historian John Haller, Jr. examines the events and circumstances which influenced the establishment and decline of 13 physio-medical colleges in the United States between 1836 and 1911, when the last college closed. He combined institutional histories with sociopolitical analysis, using a wide variety of primary sources such as contemporary professional literature, popular literature, and letters. He argues that "physio-medicals preferred ideology to the rigors of science and procrastinated when it came to building a curriculum which would include sound laboratory and clinical experiences for their students," in contrast to regular medicine which captured the title to science.

Haller considers physio-medicalism from at least four perspectives: as a distinct professional group differentiated from allopathy, homeopathy, Thomsonianism, and Eclecticism; as shaped by their 13 physio-medical colleges (in particular, the Physio-Medical Institute of Cincinnati and the Physio-Medical College of Indiana); as proponents of the "theory of vitalism" which guided "reform materia medica;" and as casualties of belated attempts to change. Primary audiences would include historians of medicine, health sciences, and preventive health care.

Haller notes that physio-medicalism (also called "sanative medicine") insisted on using only botanicals or natural drugs and emphasized the role of physicians in assisting the 'life power' or 'vital principle' in every patient. . . ." Physios demanded recognition, equal legal rights, and representation on state medical boards. As allopathic physicians and the American Medical Association consolidated their control over urban hospitals and dispensaries for clinical instruction and research, they also effectively controlled the practice and education of the physio-medicals. Physios were financially unable to meet curriculum standards set by the licensing boards, refused to purchase medicines from regular pharmacies for fear of adulteration, and objected to the use of Latin in prescription writing because of the implied secrecy. They also rejected the germ theory, the "science of probabilities," and the use of harsh/toxic chemicals (in favor of "kindly medicines"). Known as "Knights of the Lobelia Pod," they relied on at least 14 different types of preparations including infusions, extracts, lozenges, expectorants, and suppositories.

One strength of Haller's work is his interpretation of 19th-century medical practices as set within the political context of "laissez-faire" Jacksonian democracy, which allowed diverse, alternative health care practices to emerge. Although occasionally tedious in the institutional histories, the author presents a strong argument that although the physios ceased to exist as a separate profession, they contributed significantly to American health care. He notes their published advice on health and hygiene and service as primary care providers—often in rural America, among the working class.

Although Haller identifies the existence of a school of nursing at the Chicago Physio-Medical College, he neglects any further examination of nurses' roles in physio-medicalism. Discerning readers will, however, find analogies between the ideology of physios and nurses; they will notice a shared propensity toward underserved populations, and they will identify with the control exerted by allopathic medical practitioners over access to knowledge.

CYNTHIA TOMAN, RN, MSN
School of Nursing
University of Ottawa
Ottawa, Ontario, Canada K1H 8M5

Jean I. Gunn: Nursing Leader

By Natalie Riegler

(Markham, Ontario: Associated Medical Services, Inc. and Fitzhenry & Whiteside, 1997)

Jean I. Gunn was born "on the edge of an adventure." That adventure changed nursing from a vocation to a profession, and Gunn played an important role in the transformation. She entered nurses training in 1905 at the Presbyterian Hospital in New York City, under the supervision of Anna Maxwell. After working in the operating room for several years, she returned to Canada in 1913 as Superintendent of Nurses at Toronto General Hospital (TGH).

During the early 1900s, as new nursing organizations emerged in Canada, Gunn was quick to recognize their importance and to take part. As she developed professional expertise, these new associations reaped the benefits, for Gunn was a natural leader. By 1920 she was helping direct the Canadian National Association of Trained Nurses (CNATN), the Canadian Nurses' Association (CNA), the Graduate Nurses' Association of Ontario, the Canadian Association of Nursing Education, and the Canadian Red Cross Society, among others. She also served as director of the editorial board of the *Canadian Nurse Journal.* While fulfilling these many extracurricular professional obligations, Gunn met the challenges of developing her position as Superintendent of Nurses in a 735-bed hospital.

As World War I began Gunn and Shirley Wright, as officers of CNATN, submitted to the government a plan to provide volunteer-trained nurses to care for the armed forces. Their purpose was to ensure the best nursing care for soldiers and to avoid the use of untrained and unapproved nurses. The government ignored the plan, however, despite Gunn and Wright's ability to recruit trained nurses and provide additional nurses' names for service.

As supervisor of the Toronto General Hospital (TGH) School of Nursing, Gunn initiated revolutionary changes in the strict disciplinary training method generally in use. According to Riegler, she encouraged pride in her students, not servility. To encourage leadership, Gunn initiated the first student government organization in Canada at TGH. Classes elected officers and defined and enforced their own rules, and Gunn hoped that participation in student government would make for a smooth transition for the graduates into professional nursing organizations.

Nurse registration became a major issue in 1914, and Gunn was one of its greatest supporters. Registration efforts initially failed because nursing leaders refused to allow physicians to control standards, but a nurse registration act, including regulations for training schools, finally became law in 1922.

Jean Gunn's "last dream" was university education for nurses. She worked toward this goal by arranging for nurses from several schools in Toronto to meet for centralized lectures at the University of Toronto (UT) in 1918. In 1920 the Department of Public Health Nursing was established at UT, and in

1933, Gunn's long-held dream was realized with the opening of the School of Nursing at the University.

In another crusade, Gunn worked for years to obtain funding and administrative support for more graduate staff nurses at TGH. Hospital administration was finally forced to employ more graduate nurses when the New York State Board of Nurse Examiners censured TGH, threatening to cease granting legal approval to TGH graduates to work in New York hospitals. The Board strongly objected to TGH's nurse-to-patient ratio of 1 nurse to 84 patients in some areas of the hospital.

In 1934, addressing the Canadian Nurses' Association, Gunn proclaimed that the prospect of an 8-hour day had been discussed for 20 years, without action. At her urging, private-duty nurses, who were not under the authority of hospital administration, changed to an 8-hour day. By 1937 the 8-hour day was accepted for student nurses.

Throughout her impressive career, Jean Gunn received numerous honors and awards. Among these were the King's Jubilee Medal from King George V, an honorary doctorate from the University of Toronto, and the International Red Cross Florence Nightingale Medal.

Jean I. Gunn: Nursing Leader is a well-rounded history of both the woman and her profession from 1913 to 1941. Riegler has written an accessible personal history while illuminating the important issues facing nursing during this era. She provides helpful lists of Gunn's participation on committees, her leadership roles, and awards and honors, allowing the reader to gain a full perspective of Gunn's many accomplishments. References include interviews with TGH alumnae from classes between 1918 and 1946. Nurse historians will find the book an interesting, informative overview of beginning Canadian and international nursing organizations and leadership styles, and a detailed study of the power of one determined woman to bring a movement into fruition.

BONNIE L. RICHARDSON, PHD, RN
Nurse Researcher
704 Woodbury Knolls Drive
Winston-Salem, NC 27104-3488

Keeping America Sane: Psychiatry and Eugenics in the United States and Canada 1880-1940
By Ian Robert Dowbiggin
(Ithaca, N.Y.: Cornell University Press, 1997)

This book explores the thought and behavior of some pivotal figures in North American psychiatry who were associated with the eugenics movement during the period from the late 19th century to the pre-World War II era. That mental illness, mental retardation, and criminality were hereditary was unquestioned from the beginning of the asylum movement, and this belief impacted psychiatric as well as legal thought and practice well into the 20th century. In case after case, psychiatrists cited the "hereditary taint" as evidence of authentic mental illness and of diminished responsibility. Still, at the turn of the 20th century, when psychiatrists sought to base practice upon solid empirical grounds, the absence of scientific evidence for a genetic basis for these social ills led many psychiatrists to equivocate or to reject eugenics altogether.

Dowbiggin concludes that the American and Canadian psychiatrists who did advocate a hereditary cause for social ills did so for predominantly nonscientific reasons. Their individual beliefs and motivations varied, but can be characterized as related to social reform rather than scientific theory. The author points out that advocacy for legislation either permitting or, as some reformers hoped, mandating eugenic sterilization of social undesirables allowed for the exercise of psychiatric power over social policy as well as individual lives. The claim that humanitarian reform was embedded in the movement has always been suspect, but Dowbiggin credits the psychiatrist-eugenicists with being "professional men and women committed to helping those less fortunate than themselves. . . ." The eugenics movement offered an opportunity to advance the profession, for advocating psychiatric solutions to social problems was one method of legitimizing psychiatric practice outside the asylum. There is no single explanation, however, for those psychiatrists who assumed a eugenic stance.

Psychiatry has had to contend with intractable problems since the beginning of enlightenment reform. The use of reproductive control to reduce the incidence of psychiatric illness seemed a viable hypothesis even in the absence of empirical evidence to support it, and as Sir Karl Popper points out, there was an absence of compelling evidence to refute it.

Eugenics as a solution to contemporary social problems still lurks in the scientific background. Evidence from both molecular biology and the social sciences suggests that reproductive control may still be the answer to the prevention of psychiatric illness and other social problems. Dowbiggin concludes, however, that the intellectual link between eugenics and the Holocaust may insulate society from any eugenics-based solutions in the near future. Despite that acknowledged link, he rightly observes that the "spirit of eugenics is hardly crushed." We must take comfort in the knowledge that, throughout the 20th century, the great majority of psychiatrists and politicians refused to resort to eugenic solutions.

JANET COLAIZZI, PhD, RN
Professor of History and Philosophy
Saint Leo College
Tidewater Center, VA 23665

G.I. Nightingales: The Army Nurse Corps in World War II
By Barbara Brooks Tomblin
(Lexington, Ky.: The University Press of Kentucky, 1996)

Limited attention to the experiences of nurses during World War II in the literature, and the struggle of women in the military to gain recognition for their service, prompted Barbara Brooks Tomblin to pursue writing *G.I. Nightingales* in the 1970s. At the time, however, there was limited interest from publishers on the subject. That situation changed with the 50th anniversary of World War II, and renewed public interest in the era. Using information gathered from personal interviews, archival visits, and correspondence with army nurse veterans, Tomblin has created a chronological, geographical, and experiential account of nurses who served during World War II. It is apparent that she obtained prolific amounts of information during her research on army nurses. Indeed, at times, the numerous references to military units and hospitals become somewhat tedious, but helpful when presenting the military history of the war. Readers should keep in mind that this attention to detail may initially be distracting and at times confusing, but soon they will become absorbed in the unfolding story of the Army Nurse Corps during World War II.

Tomblin's account of Army nurses during World War II begins fittingly with the bombing of Pearl Harbor, Hawaii, by Japan on 7 December 1941. It follows a format focusing on activities of individual nurses before, during, and after Pearl Harbor. It then moves on to discuss the enlargement of the corps until the end of hostilities in 1945. The book follows a natural geographical organization, with each chapter focusing on a particular portion or theatre of war. For those readers not familiar with the scope of WWII, *G.I. Nightingales* will be a revelation. After reading the book one understands that the war, fought from 1941 to 1945, was truly a war that engulfed the world. Nurses served in every theatre of it, from the Middle East to Africa, the South Pacific, and Europe.

Events in each theatre of war are treated in a chronological fashion by Tomblin. She outlines the increase in the number of nurses (over 60,000 total) and military hospitals set up, and then moves them to the front lines of battle. Comments from individual nurses are scattered liberally throughout the entire text, providing an experiential focus that pulls the reader into the setting. The stories of the nurses in the Philippines are particularly moving, as they provide insight into the stark conditions under which they cared for the injured and ill while prisoners of war in a Japanese internment camp.

Tomblin provides insight into the reason for the slow progress made in the appointment of nurses as officers, originally only with relative rank, to officers holding commissioned rank and commensurate pay. She discusses the military's constant plea for more nurses and their refusal to use African American nurses until late in the war. The author also discusses how close the United States came to drafting nurses for the war, even though thousands of nurses volunteered to serve.

Although Tomblin has attempted to provide a picture of nurses' military life with meticulous detail in each theatre of war, it is provided largely within a context of dates, numbers, and military units, which at times becomes contradictory and confusing. Many readers will find themselves wanting less numerical detail but more insight into the work that army nurses performed.

This point made, Tomblin identifies the common themes that emerged from the nurses' comments. Personal characteristics such as courage, ingenuity, and an incredible work ethic, all focused on the care of young servicemen, were found among all the nurses regardless of where they served during the war. *G.I. Nightingales* is recommended for readers interested in the history of military nursing, especially for those entering military nursing service, so that they can understand the sacrifices made by a previous generation, and what their contributions mean for today's and tomorrow's military nurses.

KATHRYN M. GANSKE, MSN, RN
Adjunct Faculty
Shenandoah University
Division of Nursing
Winchester, VA 22602

Hospital Days: Reminiscence of a Civil War Nurse

By Jane Stuart Woolsey
(Roseville, Minn.: Edinborough Press, 1996)

Hospital Days records the reminiscences of Civil War nurse Jane Stuart Woolsey. Written at the conclusion of the war, the book was first published in 1868 for the family only. Although it had a limited circulation, the book found its way to a reviewer for the *New York Evening Post,* who considered it "one of the most perfect bits of English prose within our knowledge."

Woolsey and her eight siblings were raised in New York by their widowed mother. As young adults, they became absorbed in the political events that led to the Civil War. As one sister said, "When the members of the Woolsey family gave up toys, they took up politics." Deeply influenced by their mother's abhorrence of slavery, all of them were committed to abolitionism.

Eager to make a contribution to the war effort but unable to serve in the military, Woolsey and her sisters participated in the development of civilian organizations that supported the war effort. Later, under the tutelage of Katherine Wormeley and Georgeanna Woolsey, Jane studied hospital management and became the superintendent of the large barrack Union hospital established at the Fairfax Episcopal Seminary in 1863. Here she recorded the observations that later comprised this book. Characterized as compassionate with a gift for management, Woolsey was able to translate her nursing experiences into a captivating narrative describing the day-to-day work of the nurse.

Sandwiched between chapters entitled "First Days" and "Last Days," Woolsey details her concerns as superintendent with the preparation of special diets, interviewing nurse volunteers, arranging for store room supplies, and supervising work in the wards. Given the challenges of unpredictable deliveries, the "standing misunderstandings" regarding authorization of nurse procurement, an unscrupulous steward, and a profane butcher, the position of superintendent was not for the fainthearted. Woolsey responds to these trials with a mixture of zeal, humor, and empathy.

The chapter entitled, "Mail Days" testifies to the strength of Woolsey's character, her compassion, and her attention to detail. Letters arrived regularly from friends and family of the soldiers, which Woolsey found ". . . touching enough. . . . some are restrained and quiet; some are full of noble courage and patience; some are the pouring out of helpless love and sorrow. So many beg for particulars: 'Write more;' 'What did he say of *me?*'" Family members who had received word of their loved one's death wrote poignantly: ". . . I received your kind but distressing letter telling of the death of my dear son. . . . My stranger friend, I am happy to think you respected my son to take such care of him during his illness. . . ." A mother and father wrote, ". . . We felt you did all you could for our son, and more for being so kind as to write to us and let us know where are laid his mortal remains. You wrote you thought he was praising God. It was the greatest comfort to us of anything. . . . Was his mind on prayer or the Bible? He wrote to me that if he fell he should fall safe. . . . His place is vacant. . . . If you think of anything more let us know."

It is difficult to imagine someone who would not find this book fascinating reading. Woolsey's aptitude for storytelling enabled her to create a unique recollection of sensitive concern midst the atrocities of war. In sharp contrast to the current preoccupation with health care economics, *Hospital Days* offers a refreshing reminder of our distinctive nursing heritage.

SUE C. BRYANT, PHD, RN
Western Kentucky University
Associate Professor
Department of Nursing
1 Bid Red Way
Bowling Green, KY 42101

One Blood.
The Death and Resurrection of Charles R. Drew

By Spencie Love
(Chapel Hill, N.C.: University of North Carolina Press, 1996)

Myth or reality; legend or truth? Dr. Charles Drew, a pioneering researcher on the preservation of blood plasma bled to death in 1950 following injuries sustained during an auto accident. Rumors began to circulate that Dr. Drew died because he was denied medical treatment at Alamance General Hospital in Burlington, North Carolina, on account of his being Black. Many people, both Black and White, accepted these rumors as fact. The subsequent gathering of corroborating eyewitness accounts, however, reported that the hospital staff did everything they could to save Dr. Drew's life.

It was ironic that this man should have bled to death. Dr. Charles Drew entered the field of blood research in 1938 at Columbia University, where he was the first Black to receive a Doctor of Science degree in medicine in 1940. His dissertation, *Banked Blood: A Study in Blood Preservation,* and the work that followed as medical director of the Blood for Britain Project, prepared him for later challenges. He was appointed the first medical director of the American Red Cross Blood Bank, where his work contributed significantly to the supply of blood during WWII. One of the most difficult challenges he faced in this role came when the American Red Cross announced a policy that excluded Black Americans as blood donors. After three months of protests by Dr. Drew and Black citizens, the policy was changed to segregation of Black and White blood.

In 1941 Dr. Drew withdrew from the public limelight. He assumed a teaching position at Howard University Medical School and also served as chief of the department of surgery and head surgeon at Freedmen's Hospital. By 1950 Dr. Drew was the chairman of Howard University Medical School's surgery department and the chief surgeon at Freedmen's Hospital. It was in that year, traveling late at night because segregated hotel accommodations were not readily available, that Dr. Drew fell asleep at the wheel and ended up at Alamance General Hospital.

Eight months later another Black man, Maltheus Avery, was taken to the same hospital after an automobile accident. In need of neurosurgery, he was transferred to Duke Hospital in Durham, North Carolina, where he was refused treatment because no "Black beds" were available. Avery died shortly thereafter. He was also traveling at night, unable to find sleeping accommodations because of his race. Two similar stories; two different conclusions.

All this Ms. Love determined by using the techniques of investigative reporting; social, cultural, and oral history; and concepts borrowed from psychology, anthropology, and from folklore. She sets the record straight. Dr. Drew did not die because of mistreatment or neglect or from being denied a blood transfusion because of his race. He died because of the severity of his wounds. Spencie Love makes it clear that many Blacks did die because they were denied medical treatment but that Dr. Drew was not one of them. One can only speculate to what extent the Jim Crow laws contributed to the death of Mr. Avery and Dr. Drew. Ms. Love's conclusions were reached after corroborating eyewitness accounts against primary and secondary documents and news accounts. But she doesn't stop there. Intrigued with the importance of how stories shape history, and how rumors, myths, and legends are generated and perpetuated, Ms. Love's research extends beyond traditional historiography in search of important truths about a group's collective historical experience. *One Blood* refocuses Southern history.

The book brings to light the aggregate, subjective, lived experience of segregation and racial discrimination in its search for hidden clues of "traumatic historical experiences." Oral lore, passed on from generation to generation and often dismissed as "insignificant falsehoods," is gaining recognition as a method of investigating cultural heritage. Acknowledging that caution is necessary "when using oral materials as valid historical evidence—especially when no corroborating written documents are available," Ms. Love believes that, "recorders of this past will greatly expand the house of American history, opening new doors onto our increasingly complex and interrelated human story, by listening carefully to the tales, beliefs, and memories of all of America's peoples."

The contribution that *One Blood* makes to southern historiography is not the discovery of how the Drew legend developed, but the deeper exploration of legend through ". . . a prism that sheds light in more than one way. For not only does it powerfully convey the core of the black experience, it also quietly and subtly expresses the extreme tension between two clashing cultural ideals: white supremacy and democratic meritocracy." The symbolism of blood, "that blacks in this country are subject to being metaphorically bled to death," juxtaposed with Dr. Drew's mission to eliminate policies that separated Black from White blood donors and transfusions, and the loss of many lives to segregation policies in the South, carries a strong message.

The examination of cultural myths and legends in search of the subjective truth of lived experiences can have value in understanding some of the side effects of human oppression. Through the lens of legend verification, historians can more clearly understand the value of reexamining recorded history. This method of investigation can lead to expanded insights and has application for the study of nursing history. Sandra Lewenson, in *Taking Charge: Nursing, Suffrage and Feminism in America,* examines the unacknowledged earlier contributions of nursing to the suffrage movement and the larger woman's movement, contributions which have remained unnoticed by nurses, women, and society at large. The failure to record nursing's contribution to the health and well-being of society is reason enough to hold up the prism to shine new light on our history. Spencie Love's book can illuminate new ways to view nursing's story, from myth to reality, from legend to truth.

Diane J. Mancino, EdD, RN, CAE
Executive Director
National Student Nurses' Association, Inc.
Foundation of the National Student Nurses' Association, Inc.
555 West 57th St., Suite 1327
New York, NY 10019

No Time for Fear

By Diane Burke Fessler

(East Lansing: Michigan State University Press, 1996)

In *No Time for Fear* Diane Burke Fessler records oral histories of World War II nurses who served overseas in the U.S. Army, Air Force, or Navy from 1941 to 1946. She gathered information by using written questionnaires and oral interviews with almost 200 veterans, and the resulting book emphasizes the uniqueness and intensity of their wartime experiences and memories.

The nurses' recollections are clustered according to geographical and chronological divisions of the war. Fessler begins with the events of the Japanese attack on Pearl Harbor on 7 December 1941. Nurses assigned to the naval hospital at Pearl Harbor and to the naval hospital ship *USS Solace*, which was anchored in the harbor during the attack, provide fascinating descriptions of the chaos. More recollections come from nurses who were stationed at Army base hospitals on Oahu. In addition to vividly describing the attack, these nurses depict the severity of the injuries witnessed and the care provided to the thousands of injured military personnel.

Subsequent chapters progress through the battle theatres of the war. Navy nurses serving in Pacific fleet hospitals, naval medical air evacuation services, and the naval hospital ships *USS Solace* and *USS Refuge* relive their wartime experiences. Army nurses who worked in medical evacuation services, hospitals, and aboard the Army hospital ship *USS Dogwood* share the details of their similar military experiences. As one might imagine, riveting details of their contact with the enemy characterize the recollections of Army and Navy nurses imprisoned by the Japanese in the Philippines. A small group of military nurses who were stationed in China, Burma, India, Alaska, Russia, Iceland, Liberia, Brazil, and the Aleutian Islands describe their unusual posts and the work done there.

The section on wartime nursing in the European theatre is heavily represented by the recalled experiences of Army nurses. These include transcribed memories of nurses who served in England, France, North Africa, the Mediterranean, and postwar occupied Germany. There is a concentrated focus on reminiscences of Army nurses who worked at the 166th General Hospital in Le Mans, France, following the Allied invasion of Normandy. They describe in detail their basic military training, mobilization sailing to Europe, the difficult living and working conditions of a mobile tent hospital, the use of military hospital trains to evacuate the wounded, and the challenges of caring for German prisoners-of-war.

The final recollections in *No Time for Fear* depict the end of the Second World War with the victories in Europe and the Pacific. Nurses recall their experiences with the closure of overseas hospitals, the persistent issue of segregation in the military, the provision of care to both enemy and Allied prisoners-of-war, demobilization, and their difficult readjustment to civilian life.

Throughout the book, certain themes emerge from the recollections of both Army and Navy nurses. Patriotism and adventure were major reasons for choosing military duty. Many nurses describe how naïve they were in their initial understanding of the realities of war, and how initial basic military training provided minimal orientation to wartime nursing. They found living and working conditions to be primitive and harsh, especially the Army nurses serving overseas, and their rough working conditions were further complicated by limited supplies. The severity of battle injuries was shocking, often promoting a sense of helplessness and inadequacy among the nurses. In the face of massive casualties both Army and Navy nurses found it necessary to take on additional duties and medical tasks. They were often too busy providing care to the injured to look after their own safety. A sense of purpose and group identity, accompanied by humor and flexibility, enabled the nurses to sustain themselves and others throughout the war. Shared hardships forged a sisterhood. The intensity of their wartime experiences also contributed to their difficulties in readjusting to civilian life after discharge.

The strength of Fessler's work lies in her significant use of primary data obtained from a large number of World War II nurse veterans. The similarities noted among the nurses, despite serving in different branches of service and duty stations, emphasize the unique aspects of overseas wartime nursing. The recollections are vivid and compelling, leading the reader back 50 years into the events of World War II. One limitation of the book is its overrepresentation of Army nurses in comparison to those who served in the Navy. The chapters on the Pacific theatre would have been stronger had they included more recollections of naval nurse veterans. The author did not reveal her method of subject selection, and the reviewer acknowledges the possibility that Navy veterans may have been fewer or unwilling to participate in the project. She also recognizes that significantly more Army nurses were deployed overseas than their Navy counterparts. *No Time for Fear* would also have benefited from the perceptions and memories of physicians, medics, and corpsmen who worked alongside these nurses, as well as the impressions of patients who received their care.

Fessler does not provide any analysis of the nurses' experiences, and while their stories speak eloquently of the experience of war, a historian's perspective and commentary would have added much to the book. But even lacking that, *No Time for Fear* is a valuable resource. The number of surviving World War II nurse veterans is dwindling rapidly, and any attempt to document their unique experiences is important to the history of American nursing. They served in unprecedented numbers and in closer proximity to battle than ever before in American warfare. These fascinating memories will be of interest to nurses and non-nurses alike, and should lead to an increased appreciation for nurses' participation in the Second World War.

Patricia A. Connor, RN, CS, MSN
Lt. Commander, Nurse Corps, US Naval Reserve
PhD Candidate
School of Nursing
University of Virginia
Charlottesville, VA 22901

Caring and Curing:
Health and Medicine in the Western Religious Traditions
Edited by Ronald Numbers and Darrel Amundsen
(Baltimore: Johns Hopkins University Press, 1986)

Contemporary health care professionals understand that health care, science, and religion are inextricably connected. As Rosenberg (1992) cogently observed, the methods of naming and treating sickness, as well as attitudes toward the meaning of illness and the efficacy of treatment are closely linked to how groups perceive and understand their world. Disease is a biological event, but also a generation and culture-specific repertoire of verbal constructs that reflect intellectual, cultural, and institutional histories (Rosenberg & Golden, 1992). Other scholars have observed that issues related to health care, such as life style, sexuality, abortion, suicide, and euthanasia, are influenced by the social and cultural context, which includes religious beliefs.

The editors of this book collected 20 essays from established American scholars who examined various "western" religions and asked the question: how do the long, deep, entangling roots of different faith traditions shape perceptions of disease, health-seeking behaviors, disease treatments, use of resources, and health care technology development? Numbers and Amundsen maintain that both Jews and Christians have long stressed the importance of caring for the human body. For example, the Talmud went so far as to prohibit Jews from living in a city in which there was no physician, and the Puritan divine Cotton Mather ministered to bodies as well as souls in order to enhance "angelical conjunction"—the joining of spiritual and physical healing. In addition, the authors point out that the ranks of cleric-physicians included some of the most prominent pioneers in the annals of early American church history: John Clarke, one of the Baptist founders of Rhode Island; Francis Makemie, who helped bring Presbyterianism to America; Henry Melchior Muhlenberg, the patriarch of American Lutheranism; and Samuel Seabury, the first bishop of the Protestant Episcopal Church of the United States of America. Moreover, at least three denominational founders devoted part of their time to healing the sick. John Wesley, the father of Methodism, established several medical dispensaries and wrote one of the most popular medical manuals of his time. Mary Baker Eddy practiced both homeopathy and a form of mesmerism before creating the Christian Science church. Ellen White, the Seventh-day Adventist prophetess, administered hydropathic treatments to family friends and founded a chain of sanitariums. And, of course, Florence Nightingale created the secular version of the Kaiserwerth deaconesses with the establishment of professional nursing for lay women. Such examples support the editors' argument that for centuries medicine and religion have been tightly intertwined in the lives of most Christians and Jews.

The 20 chapters create a survey of health and healing of the following western religious traditions: Jewish, Early Christian, Medieval Catholic, Roman Catholic, Eastern Orthodox, Lutheran, Reformed, Anglican, Anabaptist, Baptist, Wesleyan-Methodist, Unitarian, Disciples of Christ, Mormon,

Christian Science, Adventist, Jehovah's Witness, Evangelical-Fundamental, Pentecostal, and Afro American. Each essay is a finely crafted historical narrative which explores the multifaceted relationship between health, medicine, science, and the western religious traditions. Although each author approached his topic distinctively, the chapters generally follow a chronological frame which describes and analyzes the tenets, deeds, beliefs, and practices that each of the religious traditions associates with health, wellness, healing, disease, and illness.

Taken together, the essays constitute an impressive discussion of the diffuse but pervasive presence of religion in modern life. While the book is now over a decade old, it serves as a good resource for educators and students at the baccalaureate, master's, and doctoral level. Each chapter is easily understood by nonspecialists, and should be of considerable interest not only to religious historians but to all health care professionals who must make sense of the general public's attitudes toward the proper care of the human body and the health of the soul.

Reference

Rosenberg, C., & Golden, J. 1992. *Framing Disease: Studies in Cultural History.* New Jersey: Rutgers University.

DIANE HAMILTON, PhD, RN
Associate Professor
Western Michigan University
School of Nursing
Kalamazoo, MI 49009

INDEX

American nursing, 3–4

Appalachia, 158

diagnosis, 3–5, 7, 10, 14, 17–29

Canada, 110

clinical practice, 117, 132, 133–134

early twentieth century, 10, 16–17

epidemiology, 144

hospitals, 157, 159–165

industrialization, 157, 165

influenza, 143–150, 153, 154

late nineteenth century, 10–11

miners, 157–165

nursing education, 71–73, 82–83, 84–87, 90

nursing in remote regions, 95–96, 110

obstetric nursing, 117–118, 120, 122, 126, 129, 132

occupational therapy, 39–43, 45–50, 52–53, 59–63, 64

occupied Japan, 71

pandemic, 144, 147, 149

progressive era, 118, 119

Québec, 95–98, 101, 104–105, 107, 109–110

rehabilitation, 39, 57, 63

Slagle, Eleanor Clark , 39, 41, 43, 45–50, 54, 57–64

technology, 3–5, 10, 16–17, 19–20, 22, 24, 26–28

Tracy, Susan E., 39, 41, 49–56, 61–63

training schools, 161, 163–164

wages/salaries, 169–175, 179

women's labor history, 170–171, 175–176

women's reform movement, 39, 41–43, 45–49, 51–54, 57, 63–65

Springer Publishing Company

My Fifty Years in Nursing
Give Us To Go Blithely
Doris Schwartz, RN, FAAN

"Let cheerfulness abound with industry . . . on our business all this day. Bring us to our resting beds weary and content . . . and grant us in the end the gift of sleep."

-Robert Louis Stevenson

Few books convey the excitement and wide range of opportunities possible in a nursing career as well as Doris Schwartz's vivid memoirs of her long career as a pioneering public health and geriatric nurse. She brings readers from the tenements of Brooklyn, where her patients ranged from Italian Immigrants to Mohawk Indians; to the U.S. Army, where she spent part of her time as head nurse of an amputee ward and on a floating hospital in the Pacific Ocean; to Sweden, where Schwartz visited her rural patients by bicycle; to the Frontier Nursing Service in rural Kentucky, where many patients could only be reached by horseback. Schwartz went on to Cornell University, and later the University of Pennsylvania, where she spent many satisfying years as a nurse educator, researcher, and writer. This book is informative and inspiring reading for practicing nurses and those considering a career in nursing.

Contents:
- From Where You Are to Where You Need to Be
- The Army Nurse Corps in World War II
- Public Health Nursing in Sweden
- The Frontier Nursing Service
- The Cornell-Navajo Field Health Program
- The Verb "To Wonder"
- The World Health Organization's "Expert Committee on Nursing"
- The Nurse as Primary Practitioner
- New Girl at School
- To the Great Wall of China

Nurse's Book Society Selection
1995 216pp. 0-8261-8920-2 *hard* *$28.95 (outside U.S. $33.80)*
www.springerpub.com

536 Broadway, New York, NY 10012-3955 • (212) 431-4370 • Fax (212) 941-7842